Lung Cancer

A Guide to Diagnosis and Treatment

Walter Scott, M.D.

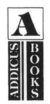

Addicus Books
Omaha, Nebraska

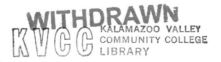

An Addicus Nonfiction Book

ISBN 1-886039-43-7
Cover design by Del Lamont, Desktopmiracles.com
Typography by Linda Dageforde
Illustrations by Bob Hogenmiller and Jack Kusler

This book is not intended to serve as a substitute for a physician, nor does the author intend to give medical advice contrary to that of an attending physician's.

Library of Congress Cataloging-in-Publication Data
Scott, Walter J., 1954-
    Lung cancer : a guide to diagnosis and treatment / Walter J. Scott.
        p. cm.
    Includes index.
        ISBN 1-886039-43-7
        1. Lungs—Cancer—Popular works. I. Title.
    RC280.L8 S36 2000
    616.99'424—dc21

                                                                00-008028

Addicus Books, Inc.
P.O. Box 45327
Omaha, Nebraska 68145
Web site: www.AddicusBooks.com

Printed in the United States of America
10 9 8 7 6 5 4 3 2

*For Christine
and for my parents*

Contents

Acknowledgments

This book would not have been possible without the efforts of a great many people. Most importantly, I wish to express my gratitude to the patients and their families. Their willingness to share their lives with me has been a source of inspiration and renewal. I also wish to thank the members of the Creighton University Multidisciplinary Chest Tumor Clinic as well as the staff of the Creighton Cancer Center for their commitment to improving the care of patients with lung cancer. Thanks also to the medical students, residents, and fellows for their hard work and tough questions.

I am grateful for the support of Rod Colvin and Susan Adams of Addicus Books. Their patience and guidance throughout the preparation of the manuscript have resulted in a much more useful book. Thanks also to James Mailliard, M.D. for his review of the chapter on chemotherapy; to Holly Adams, MSW for her review of the chapter on end-of-life care; to Albert Frank, M.D. for help with the radiation oncology chapter; and to Rose Tselentis, R.N., Thoracic Oncology Program Coordinator.

None of this would have been possible without the daily assistance of Sandra Nichols. Finally, special thanks go to Christine Beardmore, MA, my wife who is also a psychotherapist, for her work on the chapters on emotional support and complementary and alternative medicine.

Introduction

If you are reading this book, you or someone you care about has probably been diagnosed with lung cancer. Your initial reaction may have been shock, or the dread that comes with having your worst fears confirmed. You may have felt guilty, or angry, or you may have asked yourself, "Why me?" These are all normal feelings. You have a right to feel them. After surviving the initial diagnosis, you've likely found yourself pondering the inevitable question: "What happens next?"

Patients and family members often tell me that, after their diagnosis, the sheer number of tests, procedures, and treatment options overwhelms them. In writing this book, I hope to answer questions you might have about your treatment. Once you have been diagnosed with lung cancer, your survival and your quality of life depend on understanding your options and making sure that you receive the best available therapy.

Don't feel as though you have to face this alone. For one thing, according to the U.S. Center for Health Statistics, 171,500 people were newly diagnosed with lung cancer in the United States in 1998. Second, it is becoming more common for lung cancer specialists to care for these people. Third, a growing advocacy movement is arising among those living with lung cancer and their loved ones. They disseminate information about the latest therapies, advocate increased funding for lung cancer research, and promote awareness of and support for those living with lung cancer.

Thanks to new treatments and new combinations of treatments, thousands of men and women survive lung cancer each year. My wish is that this book will help you seek the best possible treatment so that you can improve your chances of becoming one of the lung cancer survivors.

1

The Lungs and Lung Cancer

The lungs are marvelously constructed organs. They deliver life-giving oxygen to every cell in our bodies. Located in the chest cavity, the lungs are composed of spongy tissue that is capable of expanding as we breathe. Each lung is divided into *lobes*. The right lung has three lobes—upper, middle, and lower. The left lung has two lobes—upper and lower.

When we inhale, air is delivered to the lungs through the *bronchial tree*. This structure consists of the windpipe or *trachea,* which branches out into two *bronchi,* one to each lung. The two bronchi further branch out into tree-like *bronchial tubes* inside the lungs. At the end of the bronchial tubes are some 300 million microscopic air sacs or *alveoli.*

The center of the chest, between the lungs, is called the *mediastinum.* This part of the chest contains the heart, and blood vessels, lymph nodes, and the esophagus. The *pulmonary arteries* and *veins* carry blood to and from the lungs. The lymph nodes, part of the immune system, are located along the breathing passages, both in the mediastinum and inside the lungs. The

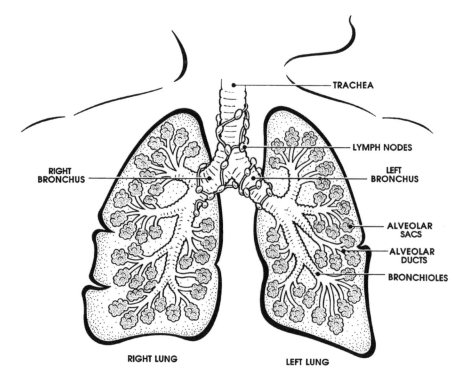

Lungs and Bronchus

esophagus, or swallowing tube, connects the mouth to the stomach.

What Is Lung Cancer?

Lung cancer is a collection of cells growing out of control in one or both lungs. It may start in one lung and spread to the other. To better understand how lung cancer forms, let's first look at how cells grow and divide. Our cells are constantly growing.

Each cell in our bodies contains a set of instructions, like software in a computer, that regulate cell behavior. Sometimes a change, or *mutation,* occurs in a cell's growth pattern. When mutations continue to occur—as many as ten to twenty may be required—the once-normal cells begin to grow abnormally. These new growths are called cancers.

Lung cancers usually arise from the cells that line the airways called *bronchial basal epithelial cell*s and the nearby mucous glands or *submucosal gland cells*. These cells are directly exposed to toxins we inhale. The transformation of normal cells into cancer begins with *hyperplasia,* which is an increase in the number of cells lining one part of the bronchial tree. This is followed by *dysplasia*, an increase in the number of abnormal lining cells. Next emerge malignant cells, or *carcinoma in situ*, which have not yet deeply invaded the tissue. Finally, the invasive cancer emerges.

Medical scientists are beginning to understand the changes that occur at the genetic and molecular levels during transformation of a normal cell into a cancer cell. They hope to learn enough to identify people at high risk of developing lung cancer and to initiate preventive therapy before it develops.

People with lung cancer aren't offered the support that those with other types of cancer receive. Attitudes towards helping are a lot less because many feel the cancer patient brought it on themselves by smoking, but that isn't always the case.

Betty, 50
Patient Advocate

Causes of Lung Cancer

Most experts believe that more than 80 percent of all cancers occur in response to environmental factors. The remaining cases are believed to arise spontaneously, as random mistakes within a

Cellular Changes

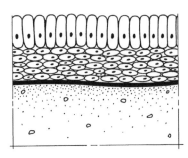

Normal Cells

These layers of cells make up the airways in the lungs. These normal cells are similar in shape and grow in an orderly fashion.

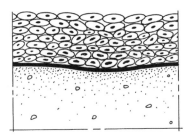

Early Changes

Here, the top layer of cells are flattened, becoming squamous cells. The change in cell structure can be caused by pollutants such as tobacco smoke.

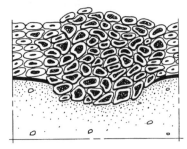

Cancer

The underlying cells change into cancer cells. They grow rapidly and form a mass which invades and destroys surrounding tissue.

cell's "software," or as a result of a set of "bad instructions" in our cells, inherited from ancestors.

Environmental factors such as smoke, toxic chemicals, radiation, oxygen-free radicals, some viruses, and even stress may cause cancer. These agents may damage a cell's instructions directly or may impair the body's immune system, the body's mechanism for fighting infections and destroying malignant cells.

Risk Factors

Smoking

Science has determined that the chemicals in cigarette smoke cause more than 80 to 90 percent of all lung cancers. Those with prolonged and heavy exposure to tobacco smoke are at high risk of developing lung cancer. The risk increases significantly with ten to twenty years of regularly smoking one to two packs of cigarettes per day.

Although less than 20 percent of significant smokers will develop lung cancer, smoking still takes a toll on the human body in other ways. Many thousands who do not develop lung cancer instead develop, and die prematurely from, illnesses such as emphysema, chronic obstructive pulmonary disease, peripheral vascular disease, stroke, and accelerated hardening of the coronary arteries, which may lead to heart attacks.

Having cancer changes one's perspective on life, usually for the better. People develop a greater appreciation for life, their relationships grow stronger and they are thankful for being alive, even if they have long-term side effects.

Robert, 46
Oncologist

Quitting smoking decreases one's risk of lung cancer. After ten years, the risk drops by half. The harmful effects of smoking on the heart also decrease immediately with smoking cessation.

Before 1930, the federal government kept few statistics on lung cancer because the disease was so rarely seen. However, by

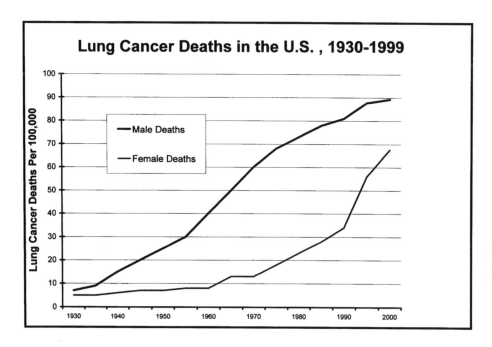

American Cancer Society

1986, it had long been the leading cause of cancer deaths in American men, and it had surpassed breast cancer as the leading cause of death from cancer in American women. This increase in lung cancer among women is particularly alarming. Statistics show a 150 percent increase in lung cancer in women from 1974 to 1994, compared to only a 20 percent increase for men. How did lung cancer become the most common cause of death from cancer in both sexes in just sixty years? The rise in cigarette consumption is the reason.

Age

Increasing age lowers one's defenses to virtually all diseases. Lung cancer is unusual, but not unheard of, in persons younger than forty.

Heredity

Family history plays a role as well. Although there does not seem to be a specific gene or class of genes associated with lung cancer, there does seem to be a genetic predisposition involving many types of genes in combination. Therefore, having a number of relatives with lung cancer may mean that one is predisposed to develop cancer if he/she engages in risky behavior such as smoking.

Environmental Pollution

Other environmental factors are thought to increase the risk of lung cancer. *Asbestos*, a fibrous material once commonly used in the construction of homes and other buildings, is considered a *carcinogen*, a cancer-causing chemical. Asbestos fibers may break into particles and float into the environment. When inhaled, they may stick to the lungs. For those exposed to asbestos and tobacco smoke, the risk of lung cancer is three to four times greater. *Radon*, an odorless gas created by the radioactive decay of uranium, is also considered a carcinogen. Found in soil and rocks, radon may seep into homes. Other chemicals that increase the risk of lung cancer include nickel, vinyl chloride, arsenic, and chromium.

> *My friends acted awkward toward me after my lung cancer diagnosis. They didn't know what to say or do. Just be there to listen and help someone stay involved in life.*
>
> *Bob, 36*
> *Patient*

9

It's important to note that the presence of more than one of these factors increases a person's risk even further.

Types of Lung Cancer

There are more than a dozen types of lung cancer, but about 90 percent fall into two main categories: *small cell* and *non-small cell*. The two forms of cancer grow and spread differently and are treated differently. The type is determined according to the size and other characteristics of the cancer cells as they appear under a microscope.

Small Cell Lung Cancer

About 20 to 25 percent of all lung cancers fall into this category. Small cell is often found in secretory cells that line the major breathing tubes. Small cell tends to grow more quickly. It has often spread to the lymph nodes in the center of the chest by the time of diagnosis, and may even have spread through the bloodstream, to other places in the body.

Non-Small Cell Lung Cancer

Seventy to 80 percent of all lung cancers fall into this category. Non-small cell lung cancer grows slower than small cell and is more often confined to the chest when it is first diagnosed. There are several forms of non-small cell lung cancer.

Squamous cell carcinomas are typically found in the larger airways inside the lung. The tumors are generally more centrally located in the chest than other cancers. They are the most common lung cancers in men and comprise about 30 percent of all lung cancers.

Adenocarcinomas are found in the mucous glands that line the airways. They are often located toward the edges of the lungs. Sometimes, in reviewing old chest x-rays, it seems adenocarcinomas have arisen at the site of old scars inside the lungs. These cancers are sometimes called *scar carcinomas.* Adenocarcinomas make up about 40 percent of all lung cancers.

Large cell carcinomas usually have larger cells than other lung cancers and typically form near the outer edges of the lungs. They often start in the smaller breathing tubes and may spread rapidly. They comprise about 10 percent of all lung cancers.

There are several remaining types of non-small cell lung cancer including several uncommon types. These include *bronchoalveolar carcinoma,* which appears in the microscopic air sacs within the lungs. It is a slower-growing cancer, appearing most frequently in older adults.

2

Symptoms of Lung Cancer

Many symptoms of lung cancer resemble symptoms of other common conditions. Accordingly, a physician will consider any symptoms of lung cancer in the context of a patient's health background—age, smoking history, occupational exposure, and family history.

For example, the chance that a symptom is caused by lung cancer in a 25-year old woman who never smoked is very small. By contrast, the same symptom in a 65-year-old woman who has smoked two packs of cigarettes per day over the past forty-two years is likely the result of lung cancer until proven otherwise.

The symptoms of lung cancer may be divided into three main groups. The first group is caused by cancer growing in the lungs. The second group arises when lung cancer grows outside of the lung into nearby parts of the chest. The third group indicates that the cancer has spread beyond the chest and into other parts of the body, a condition known as *metastasis*.

Symptoms of Cancer in the Lung

Persistent Coughing

Lung cancers arise from the cells lining the airways. The nerves lining the airways detect the presence of anything foreign—dust, dirt, blood, or tumor. These nerves stimulate the cough reflex, designed to help the body rid itself of particles and keep the airways clean. If a tumor develops in the large airways, cough may be a prominent symptom. Cough is present in anywhere from 20 to 80 percent of cases diagnosed. Patients with lung cancer who never complain of cough probably have tumors located away from the center of the lung, in the smaller airways, where cough receptors are few.

> *I first went to the doctor with wheezing. X-rays then showed a tumor in my lung. Fortunately, it was an early stage cancer, and I could have surgery.*
> *Elizabeth, 69*
> *Patient*

Coughing Up Blood

If the surface of a tumor bleeds, the patient may cough up blood-tinged mucous. This serious symptom, *hemoptysis,* should be evaluated immediately.

Wheezing

A tumor may result in *wheezing,* the sound produced when air tries to pass through a partially blocked airway in the lung. Remember, a tumor will produce *localized wheezing* best heard on the side of the chest where the tumor is located.

Coughing Dark Sputum

When breathing passages are blocked completely, infection may occur in the blocked or obstructed area. This leads to fevers and coughing up dark *sputum.* It is not to be confused with the infection from pneumonia, which responds to antibiotic treatment.

Symptoms of Cancer Spreading into the Chest

Chest Pain

The surface lining of the lungs (*visceral pleura*) and the inside lining of the chest cavity (*parietal pleura*) are supplied with many nerve fibers. Therefore, a cancer that irritates the surface of the lung or the chest wall without growing into it can cause *chest pain.* The pain usually occurs where the cancer is irritating the pleura. It may be constant or it can come and go with breathing. This is called *pleuritic chest pain.* It suggests that the cancer may be growing on the surface of the lung and even into the chest wall. If the cancer has invaded the surface of the lung or the chest wall, it is more advanced. However, sometimes the cancer may irritate the surface of the lung without actually growing into it. Often surgery is the only way to find out exactly how far the cancer has spread.

I've worked with lung cancer patients for about 10 years, and one thing continues to amaze me—the strength of the human spirit. It can withstand all the confusion that is put into one's life.

Tim, 44
Pulmonary Rehabilitation Specialist

Because lung tissue itself has no nerves that sense pain, cancer may grow to a large size within the lung without causing pain. This is one reason why lung cancer is difficult to diagnose in its early stages.

Persistent Hoarseness

The *laryngeal nerves* supply the vocal cords and allow them to move, giving us our normal voice. These nerves start in the head, travel down into the chest, and then go back up into the neck to supply the voice box and vocal cords. Lung cancer may grow into one of these nerves where it passes through the chest. If this happens, the vocal cord supplied by the nerve becomes weakened or even paralyzed, and a person becomes hoarse. Persistent hoarseness or a change in the quality of one's voice needs to be evaluated. A chest x-ray should be obtained as part of this evaluation.

Drooping Eyelid

If the cancer involves the sympathetic nerves, one of the eyelids may droop slightly or take longer to open than the other (*lid lag*). The sympathetic nerves, which control such involuntary actions as breathing, run in a chain on either side of the spine. These nerves are most vulnerable to damage from cancer arising in the top of the lungs. Because the chest cavity narrows in this area, a growing cancer may easily compress and grow into the surrounding structures.

Shortness of breath had become part of my life. I was weak from losing 20 pounds over three years. At first, doctors found only an infection. I thought it was cancer all along, and it was. Seek an accurate diagnosis.

Phyllis, 57
Patient

A person may also have trouble seeing because one pupil is dilated (*miosis*), or may notice that one side of the face is drier, that it doesn't become sweaty (*anhidrosis*). A combination of these symptoms is called *Horner's syndrome.*

Pain in the Arm and Arm Pit

Constant pain in the armpit and the arm, often associated with other symptoms, is known as *Pancoast's syndrome.* The nerves that supply the arm come from the neck and travel over the top of the lung. A lung cancer in this area may compress these nerves, causing severe pain.

Shortness of Breath

Also called *dyspnea,* shortness of breath is a common symptom among patients with lung cancer. Lung cancers may cause shortness of breath in many ways. A tumor that arises in a major airway and blocks the passage of air into an entire lung may cause shortness of breath. Fluid that builds up around the outside of a lung in response to the cancer, a *pleural effusion,* may occupy so much space within the chest cavity that the lung cannot fully expand. Lung cancer may even affect the sac around the heart, the *pericardium.* It may cause fluid to build up within the sac, preventing the heart from working properly and producing shortness of breath. Finally, shortness of breath can also be caused by damage to the phrenic nerves, found in the diaphragm, a muscle important to breathing. If lung cancer involves one of these nerves, the half of the diaphragm that it supplies becomes paralyzed. Movement of air in and out of the chest decreases, causing a shortness of breath.

> *Surround yourself with positive people. I remember a patient who got so tired of having to pick up everyone's spirits that she finally put a sign on the door that read: "Optimists Only."*
>
> *Cynthia, 26*
> *Nurse*

Swelling of the Face or Arms

Lung cancer arising in the right lung is most likely to compress the *superior vena cava*, the great vein that drains the blood from the head and arms and delivers it back to the heart and lungs. This compression results in swelling of the face and arms, or *superior vena cava syndrome*. This may prove serious if swelling in the neck and trachea interferes with breathing.

Symptoms of Cancer Spreading Beyond the Chest

Lung cancer spreads when cancer cells break off from the main or primary lung cancer, entering the bloodstream and traveling to other places in the body. Symptoms caused by metastasis may be the first ones that a patient reports to the doctor.

Neurological Symptoms

When lung cancer spreads to the central nervous system, the brain and spinal cord, *headache* may occur. At first they may seem no different than common tension headaches. Only when headaches persist or become more severe do most patients seek evaluation. Other neurological symptoms include changes in *alertness* as well as *nausea* and v*omiting* not related to another cause. Less common symptoms include *weakness*, either generalized or in the extremities, *loss of bowel or bladder control*, and *seizures*.

I moved in with my godmother when she was diagnosed with lung cancer. We had a nightly ritual of watching Leave It to Beaver, Donna Reed and Talk Soup. It made us laugh and gave us some great memories. She has been cancer free for seven years.

Laura, 33
Friend of Patient

17

Skeletal Pain

When lung cancer spreads to bone, it destroys the adjacent bone as it grows, causing pain. Localized skeletal pain in someone suspected of having lung cancer should therefore be evaluated with additional tests to determine if a metastasis is present. The most common sites for bone metastases are in the spine, the pelvic bones, and the femur, the large bone in the thigh.

Nonspecific symptoms

Nonspecific symptoms may have many causes. If these symptoms are noted in a person suspected of having lung cancer, the disease may have spread to areas beyond the chest.

Significant *weight loss*—a decrease of 10 percent or more of a person's usual weight—is one such symptom. While the exact cause of weight loss in this situation is not known, it seems to correlate with the amount of tumor present in the body. The amount of tumor, in turn, correlates with the likelihood of a distant metastasis being present. Poor appetite (*anorexia*) may occur for similar reasons. *Fatigue* may also be a symptom of advanced lung cancer. These same nonspecific symptoms may also occur during treatment for lung cancer. Patients should alert the healthcare professionals about symptoms that arise during treatment.

3

Diagnosing Lung Cancer

Some patients show signs of lung cancer during a physical examination. Other times, patients show no obvious signs, and the presence of lung cancer comes as a surprise to both doctor and patient. In fact, in up to 20 percent of cases, lung cancer is suspected only after a routine x-ray.

A true diagnosis can be made only upon the completion of diagnostic tests. If, upon the completion of a thorough physical examination, a doctor suspects lung cancer, he/she may order from a number of tests that will confirm the presence of cancer and the extent of any spread.

Diagnostic Tests

Chest X-Ray

An ordinary chest x-ray is still the most common imaging study performed whenever symptoms or physical examination suggest disease in the chest. The discovery of a mass in the lung is the most common chest x-ray finding in a patient with lung cancer. The chest x-ray may also detect an abnormal widening of the area between the lungs. Such an abnormal contour may indicate the presence of a tumor or lymph nodes that have enlarged as the result of a tumor.

Chest x-rays may also show signs of pneumonia, fluid around the lungs, or abnormalities in the bones. Comparison of old chest x-rays with more recent ones allows doctors to estimate the growth of a tumor. If a tumor has not grown or changed as shown by chest-rays obtained over at least a two year period, the chance of the tumor being a cancer is less than 5 percent.

People are initially shocked with the diagnosis. Feelings of disbelief, denial and anger are common. There is no right or wrong way to cope; everyone progresses through emotions differently.

Chris, 40
Counselor

Computerized Tomography

The *computerized tomography (CT) scan*, also known as a *computerized axial tomography (CAT) scan,* of the chest is standard for evaluating patients with known or suspected lung cancer. A CT scan produces cross-sectional images or "slices" of the body. A chest CT provides more detail and information than a chest x-ray. It can confirm the presence of a tumor first seen on a chest x-ray, and can better identify characteristics of the tumor, such as calcification or an irregular surface. Further, a chest CT is much more accurate than a chest x-ray at identifying enlarged lymph nodes in the lung or in the center of the chest. This is important because enlarged lymph nodes may contain metastatic lung cancer cells. Studies suggest that a chest CT may also aid early detection of lung cancer in high-risk patients.

Positron Emission Tomography

The *positron emission tomography (PET)* is an imaging test similar to x-rays and CT scans; however, PET scans reveal the function of cells, whereas the other tests show only cell structure. A patient undergoing a PET scan will first be given a sugar solution intravenously. In the case of lung cancer, cancer cells use sugar, or *glucose*, at a faster rate than normal. If cancer is present in a lung, a tumor will show up in a PET scan, having absorbed the sugar solution. The more glucose it takes up, the more likely it is a cancer. Studies suggest that PET is highly accurate at predicting whether a tumor is a cancer.

Sputum Cytology

Cytology refers to the study of cells. Testing the cellular makeup of sputum involves collecting mucous coughed up and examining it under the microscope to look for malignant cells. The most accurate way to perform this test is to collect early-morning samples on three separate days.

> *When I was first diagnosed, it was hard for me to believe it. I was stunned. But as the reality sunk in, I was determined to fight the disease.*
>
> *Betty, 59*
> *Patient*

Biopsies

Imaging studies can reveal important features about tumors, but cannot provide absolute proof that a cancer is present. Such a determination can be made only with a tissue analysis. This means doing a *biopsy*, gathering a tissue sample from the tumor. A physician will choose from several methods to perform a biopsy, depending on such factors as the likelihood that cancer is present and the size and location of the tumor.

Bronchoscopy

This procedure allows a physician to look inside the lung with a tube called a *bronchoscope*. Since cancers often arise inside the airways, a specialist performing the *bronchoscopy* can often see a tumor located in the large air passages of the lungs and can then biopsy it to determine if it is a cancer. The test provides helpful information about the location and stage of the tumor and whether it can be completely removed with surgery. Bronchoscopy, though, is less successful in examining tumors farther out, toward the edges of the lung.

> *My 30-year-old friend was diagnosed with lung cancer. She didn't expect to live long enough to see her son born. She just saw him turn five!*
>
> *Mary, 39*
> *Friend of a Survivor*

Bronchoscopy can be performed without putting patients to sleep. Patients sometimes cough, but generally tolerate the procedure well.

Transthoracic Needle Aspiration (TTNA)

A *transthoracic needle aspiration* (*TTNA*) is another common method used to obtain a sample of a tumor. The test is usually performed by a radiologist. After injecting a local anesthetic, the radiologist uses an x-ray machine to guide a needle through the chest wall and into the tumor. Cells from the tumor are sucked into a syringe attached to the needle. This technique is used mostly to study tumors closer to the chest wall, instead of more centrally located tumors.

A specially trained pathologist then examines the cell samples under a microscope to check for malignancy. TTNA is relatively simple for the patient, can be done as an outpatient procedure, and doesn't require a general anesthetic. TTNA can also be used to biopsy enlarged lymph nodes. The patient, however, must be able to cooperate by holding his/her breath during certain parts of the procedure.

A disadvantage of TTNA is that a certain number of patients will develop a collapsed lung (*pneumothorax*) when the needle passes through it. Most of the time, the collapsed lung simply reexpands. Sometimes a larger *chest tube* has to be placed between the ribs to expand the lung.

A more serious disadvantage is that sometimes the needle misses the part of the tumor that contains the cancer cells. The test might wrongly suggest that the tumor is benign. Still, the doctor may suspect cancer based on the size of the nodule, the patient's age, and smoking history. The physician may then order a repeat biopsy using a different method or recommend watching the nodule by getting another x-ray in several weeks. If the nodule grows, cancer may be suspected.

When one of our co-workers was diagnosed with lung cancer, we treated her just as we had before. Not showing fear and talking about it openly helped her tremendously.

Alex, 32
Physician Assistant

Cervical Mediastinoscopy

This method is occasionally used to biopsy a tumor but more often to biopsy the mediastinal lymph nodes, those toward the center of the chest. *Cervical mediastinoscopy* is a minimally invasive surgery in which a small incision is made directly over the trachea at the base of the neck, just above the breastbone. A mediastinoscope, a small tube that the surgeon looks through, is inserted along the trachea. The surgeon passes an instrument through the mediastinoscope and removes a piece of a tumor or enlarged lymph node.

A patient must first be under general anesthesia; however, the procedure may be performed on an outpatient basis. The procedure is generally very safe, but is often underused because some surgeons are reluctant to perform it. This may be due to inexperience with the technique.

Endoscopic Lymph Node Biopsy

During this procedure, an *upper gastrointestinal endoscope* is passed through the mouth and into the esophagus. Once in the correct position, a biopsy tool may be used to sample nearby lymph nodes. No incision is required, and the patient does not have to be under a general anesthetic.

> *Be proactive! Seek information. Ask questions. You should never leave the doctor with a question unanswered.*
>
> *Rosemary, 70*
> *Patient*

Video-assisted Thoracoscopy (VATS)

VATS is commonly used to perform an *excisional biopsy* of a lung tumor, but the procedure is usually possible only if the tumor is near the surface of a lung. Also called a *wedge resection,* an excisional biopsy removes the entire tumor rather than taking sample tissue, as does a needle biopsy. A minimally invasive technique, *VATS* may also be used to biopsy lung tumors and lymph nodes that may contain cancer and to perform other procedures, including the removal of a lobe of a lung or even an entire lung.

The patient must receive a general anesthetic in order to undergo VATS. A small incision is made between the ribs, where the surgeon can insert a special tube containing a small television camera. This allows the surgeon to see the inside of the chest on a television monitor. Other small incisions may be made for surgical instruments. Because the incisions are small and the ribs do not have to be spread apart, the patient generally feels less pain and recovers faster than from a standard chest incision.

Exploratory Thoracotomy

There are times when exploratory surgery using a *thoracotomy incision* must be performed to diagnose a lung tumor. This may be the case if previous attempts to diagnose a tumor with less invasive tests have failed and if doctors are highly suspicious of cancer. In this procedure the tumor is completely removed during surgery. If the medical team also discovers that the tumor is indeed a cancer, then a complete cancer operation, such as removing a lobe of the lung and affected lymph nodes, may be performed.

Always ask about the risks or complications of a test and how it compares to other tests. You may also wish to ask about the accuracy of any given test. Answers to these questions will help you and your doctor plan the best series of diagnostic tests.

> *Life is a constant source of new challenges. Lung cancer is one of them. It's not an easy challenge to face. Start by stepping into the ring with a positive attitude.*
>
> *Terry, 64*
> *Patient*

Screening for Lung Cancer

Screening for a disease such as lung cancer involves looking for it at an early stage, before it causes any symptoms. Treatment at such an early stage improves the prospects of a cure. The survival rate for patients with early stage lung cancer is better than that for patients with more advanced disease.

Large clinical trials have failed to demonstrate that screening high risk persons with frequent chest x-rays lowers overall mortality from lung cancer. Still, researchers have found that a specific imaging test, a *low-dose spiral CT scan,* is much more effective than the standard chest x-ray at detecting lung cancer, especially in an early stage. These scans can detect small abnormalities, usually nodules, which may or may not be cancerous. However, even this CT scan doesn't always tell the whole story. Abnormal findings should be evaluated by cancer specialists who may order additional tests, if necessary, to determine whether a growth is malignant.

There are a lot of support and educational opportunities out there. Unfortunately, they won't come knocking at your door. Patients must take the initiative to seek out this information.

Amber, 43
Social Worker

Since early detection with low-dose spiral CT has not yet been shown to reduce overall lung cancer mortality, the government and insurance companies do not pay for the test when it is used for screening. Nonetheless, in many parts of the country both physicians and members of the public have already accepted low-dose spiral CT as a valid screening test for lung cancer. The test is widely available since most hospitals have spiral CT scanners now and it only takes a few minutes to perform. Many hospitals and clinics are offering the test for approximately $300.

Despite its wide availability, because interpretation of the test must be done by experts, it is recommended that you undergo the test at a major medical center or university as part of a clinical trial.

4

Staging Lung Cancer

The process of determining how far a cancer has spread is called *staging.* Staging is determined by both biopsies and imaging—x-rays or scans. The staging system is used throughout the world. It allows doctors and researchers to speak one common language when devising and evaluating new treatments.

Staging is important for several reasons. The stage of the disease is the most important indicator of a person's *prognosis,* the likely outcome of a disease process. The prognosis of a person with lung cancer is spelled out in terms of five-year survival or the likelihood that the patient will be alive five years from the time of diagnosis. The stage of the disease is also a key factor in determining the kind of treatment that a patient will receive.

Staging Small Cell Lung Cancer

In most patients with small cell lung cancer, the disease has already spread to the mediastinal lymph nodes or elsewhere in the body by the time of diagnosis. Complete surgical removal of the tumor is not possible. The staging system divides patients into two main groups:

- *Limited disease (LD),* in which the cancer is limited to the chest. The cancer is found in only one lung and nearby lymph nodes. The two-year survival rate is 15 percent.
- *Extensive disease (ED)* or *advanced* stage, in which the cancer has spread beyond the chest to other parts of the body. The two-year survival rate is 2 percent.

The few patients whose small cell lung cancer is confined to the one lung are classified as having *very early stage disease.*

Organs Often Affected by Small Cell Lung Cancer

Liver

At the time of diagnosis, spread to the liver is found in up to 30 percent of patients. This may show up as an abnormal blood test of liver function. Most specialists recommend a CT scan to evaluate the liver and other sites in the abdomen.

Brain

Spread to the brain may occur in 10 to 27 percent of patients. Therefore, a CT scan of the head is routinely performed in order to image the brain.

Bone

Spread to the bone is found about 30 percent of the time during the initial evaluation. Therefore, doctors often perform a *bone scan.* It remains the most sensitive test for detection of bone metastases, even when symptoms such as bone pain are absent.

Bone Marrow

The bone marrow may also be involved 17 to 34 percent of the time. For this reason, some specialists recommend routine sampling of the bone marrow with a *bone marrow biopsy* or *bone marrow aspiration.* Others recommend bone marrow biopsy only if no other site of metastatic disease is found. In the future, *magnetic resonance imaging (MRI)* may prove to be more sensitive at detecting bone marrow metastases than a biopsy.

Staging Non-Small Cell Lung Cancer

The staging system for non-small cell lung cancer differs from that for small cell. In a significant number of patients, non-small cell lung cancer is not as widespread at the time of the initial evaluation. Therefore, a more specific system is helpful to describe how far the cancer has spread. Doctors use the TNM system.

> *Cancer treatments don't make people as sick as they used to years ago. People are much more comfortable and ready to go through aggressive therapy.*
>
> *Sheila, 42*
> *Radiation Therapist*

T is for tumor (size and extent of spreading).

N is for lymph nodes (spread to lymph nodes).

M is for metastasis (spread to other organs).

A number, from 0 to 4, is placed next to each letter, to indicate the extent of spread in that category. A 3 would indicate more spread than a 1.

Let's look at an example. The designation T1 would describe a tumor found early—the 1 is at the lower end of the scale. If there are no lymph node metastases, a 0 (zero) is added to the N, so the description reads N0. Finally, if no spread elsewhere is noted, a 0 is added to the M. So, M0 would mean no metastasis. The complete description, T1N0M0, indicates the earliest stage of non-small cell lung cancer.

Consider another example. A larger tumor may be T2, while a tumor that is growing into adjacent structures in the chest could be T3 or T4. The presence of cancer in the lymph nodes might mean the node (N) stage would be either N2 or N3, depending on which ones are affected. If the cancer has spread outside the chest, the metastatic (M) stage might be M1.

Once the TNM designation is established, a stage is assigned. The stages range from Stage I to Stage IV. (A complete table of TNM designations, as they relate to the stages of non-small cell lung cancer, is listed in the Appendix in the back of this book.)

My mother, 69, had a lung removed after her diagnosis of Stage I non-small cell lung cancer. In speaking with other patients, I was amazed at how much can be done to fight lung cancer.

Scott, 42
Son of survivor

Stages of Non-Small Cell Lung Cancer

Stage I

Cancer is found only inside the lung. It has not spread to any lymph nodes. More recently, stage I was subdivided into IA for smaller tumors and IB for larger tumors.

Stage II

Cancer is found inside the lung, but has also spread to nearby lymph nodes. More recently, stage II was subdivided into IIA for smaller tumors and IIB for larger tumors.

Stage III

Cancer has spread beyond the lung to nearby structures (chest wall or diaphragm) or to lymph nodes in the center of the chest or at the base of the neck. Stage III is subdivided into IIIA for tumors that may be treated by surgery and stage IIIB for tumors that are usually not treated by surgery.

Stage IV

Cancer has spread to other parts of the body.

Organs Often Affected by Spreading Non-Small Cell

Adrenal Glands

These small glands on top of the kidneys are one of the places to which non-small cell lung cancer typically spreads. Sometimes an enlarged adrenal gland or other evidence of metastasis in the abdomen may require confirmation with a needle biopsy.

Liver

The liver is another place to which non-small cell lung cancer frequently spreads. Chest x-rays and a CT of the chest and upper

Survival Rates for Non-Small Cell Lung Cancer

Stage	5-Year Survival Rate (%)
IA	67%
IB	57%
IIA	55%
IIB	39%
IIIA	23%
IIIB	3-7%
IV	1%

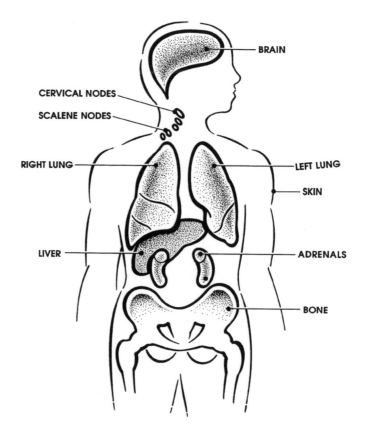

BRAIN

CERVICAL NODES

SCALENE NODES

RIGHT LUNG

LEFT LUNG

SKIN

LIVER

ADRENALS

BONE

Common Sites for Lung Cancer Metastasis

abdomen can determine spread to both the liver and the adrenal glands.

Bone

If findings suggest the possibility of metastases to bone, a bone scan should be obtained. Both an x-ray and an MRI scan of the bone may be needed to determine the extent of the spread. On rare occasions, a bone biopsy may also be necessary to make a final determination.

Brain

Neurological symptoms are further evaluated with a head CT or MRI of the brain. An MRI is a highly specialized imaging method that uses a strong magnetic field to take detailed pictures of organs and tissues. Positron emission tomography (PET) is being used by some centers to identify metastases in the brain and elsewhere in the body. Early results suggest that PET may accurately detect metastases before they produce symptoms.

Remember, staging lung cancer is important in setting up the best treatment plan. If you or a loved one has been diagnosed with lung cancer, be sure to talk to your physician about determining the stage of the disease.

5

Surgery

The goal of surgery in treating lung cancer is to remove all cancer from the body. Removing only a portion of the cancer does not improve survival and unnecessarily exposes the patient to risks related to the surgery. Therefore, doctors recommend surgery only when it seems very likely that the surgeon can remove all cancer that can be seen with the naked eye (the cancer is *resectable*) and when it is clear that the patient is strong enough to survive the operation. With modern imaging studies, doctors can more accurately estimate whether all visible cancer can be removed at the time of surgery. However, in some instances a final decision about removing the cancer can only be made after the surgeon has looked into the chest cavity.

To determine if a patient is strong enough to undergo surgery, other medical conditions must be taken into account. If the patient seems generally well, then more specific information regarding heart and lung function will be obtained. Tests of cardiovascular function help to determine if someone has the strength to undergo treatment. Health care professionals can estimate someone's exercise ability by simply asking a person to climb one or two flights of stairs while observing the breathing rate. Conducting a formal exercise treadmill test provides a more accurate estimate of exercise capacity.

Before performing an operation to remove part or all of a person's lung, a surgeon makes certain that the amount of lung remaining after the operation will be sufficient to allow the patient to live without being incapacitated. The surgeon will first want to see the results of *pulmonary function tests*. These tests evaluate lung function by measuring the amount of air that a person breathes in and out. These tests include an *arterial blood gas analysis*. This determines how well the lungs add oxygen to the blood and remove waste gases such as carbon dioxide from the blood. This involves drawing blood from an artery, most commonly the radial artery, near the wrist. The blood for most other tests are drawn from veins.

Measurement of *diffusing capacity* is another important test of lung function often performed at the time of pulmonary function testing. This test measures how well the tiny blood vessels in the lung function. Sometimes a *perfusion scan* is obtained to measure the amount of blood flowing to one lung compared to the other lung. It may help doctors decide if a person can tolerate the partial or entire removal of a lung.

Types of Surgery

Thoracotomy involves making an incision between the ribs and carefully spreading them apart to gain access to the chest. It is the most common way to operate on the lungs.

However, minimally invasive techniques allow surgeons to operate on the lungs through multiple smaller incisions and generally without spreading the ribs apart. One technique involves passing a tiny television camera attached to a special telescope, a *thoracoscope,* through a small incision into the chest. The surgeon and the other members of the surgery team view the inside of the chest on a television monitor. However, some controversy remains over the use of this technique to treat lung cancer.

Once the surgeon has gained access to the lungs, he/she performs one of several standard procedures. *Pneumonectomy* is the name for the removal of an entire lung. Removal of one lobe of a lung is called a *lobectomy.* Lobes of the lung, in turn, are made up of segments. Removing a segment is called a *segmentectomy.* Removing a nodule from any part of the lung without regard to the underlying structure is generally called a *wedge resection.* Whatever the procedure, the surgeon must remove enough lung tissue surrounding the cancer so as not to leave any cancer cells behind. The surgeon must also remove any lymph nodes that the cancer cells drained into. This generally means that the surgeon must perform at least a lobectomy and sometimes a pneumonectomy.

> *Three weeks after my lung cancer surgery, I was out playing tennis again. I had never smoked and my pulmonary tests before-hand were very good. I think your lifestyle before cancer does indicate how well you will recover.*
>
> *Sue, 42*
> *Survivor*

What Happens During Surgery?

Surgery to treat lung cancer requires a general anesthetic. Once the patient is asleep, a special breathing tube is placed through the mouth and into the windpipe. This tube is attached to a ventilator. The anesthesiologist monitors the patient carefully.

Surgery

Before operating on a lung, the surgeon may look down the breathing tube and into the breathing passages with the broncho-scope to confirm the exact location of the tumor and to make sure the cancer has not spread. In some cases, the surgeon also performs a *mediastinoscopy* to sample the lymph nodes in the center of the chest. If cancer is found in these lymph nodes, surgery is usually canceled since surgery alone is not the best treatment for such cancer. If there is no evidence of spread, the surgeon proceeds, most commonly performing a thoracotomy to gain access to the lung. Once inside, the surgeon decides whether to remove part or all of the lung based on the size and location of the tumor, evidence of spread within the chest, and further evaluation of the mediastinal lymph nodes.

After my husband had surgery to remove his lung cancer, the doctor told him to go sit on the beach and watch the pretty girls go by. That sure put some spunk back into his system.

Cecilia, 61
Wife of Survivor

Proper evaluation of the lymph nodes is crucial. Without this information, it may be impossible to know the true stage of the cancer. As mentioned earlier, the stage of the cancer determines the optimal treatment. Further, patients who do not have their lymph nodes sampled may not be eligible for certain clinical trials of state-of-the-art cancer therapy.

Still, many surgeons do not perform this part of the operation. Some believe that merely feeling the lymph nodes and noting if they are enlarged or firm is all that is neces-sary to determine if they contain cancer cells. Some or all of the mediastinal lymph nodes from several different locations must be removed so that a pathologist may examine them under the microscope. This is the only accurate way to determine whether the cancer has spread to these lymph nodes. An operation for lung cancer is not complete if the mediastinal lymph nodes have not been sampled and sent to a pathologist. Ask your surgeon if he/she plans to sample the mediastinal lymph nodes during the surgery. If not, seek a second opinion.

After the surgery, ask the doctor to explain the findings of the pathology report, including the final stage of the cancer and whether the mediastinal lymph nodes contained cancer cells.

What to Expect After Surgery

I called the American Cancer Society and surfed the web, devouring any information I could find about cancer. At a time like this, there is no such thing as having too much information or support.

Eric, 50
Husband of Patient

Removing part or all of a lung is a major operation. Patients usually spend at least a few days to a week in the hospital. Sometimes patients will spend the first day or two after surgery in an intensive care unit.

Most patients recover from the surgery without complications. Others, however, may develop complications such as wound infection or *pneumonia*. To help prevent pneumonia after lung surgery, patients should take deep breaths to keep their lungs expanded. Respiratory therapists and the medical and nursing staff can offer breathing exercises to help prevent these complications after surgery.

Understandably, it's painful to take a deep breath after chest surgery. Sometimes doctors write orders for pain medication indicating that the patient must ask for the medication before the nurse can administer it. Unfortunately, some patients are reluctant to ask, fearing that they are not being "good patients" or that they may become addicted to the pain medication. Neither fear is valid.

Remember, it's best to ask for pain medications *before* the pain starts.

Patients whose pain is well controlled will be able to take deeper breaths and will generally get well faster. Many hospitals use *patient-controlled anesthesia (PCA),* which allows the patient to simply push a button and receive pain medicine through an *intravenous* line (IV). Another method of pain control is a *thoracic epidural catheter.* With this procedure, the anesthesiologist inserts a thin tube along the back to numb the chest region. It provides very good pain relief.

At the end of an operation, the surgeon may place *chest tubes* between the ribs. These tubes drain any fluid or air from inside the chest. The chest tubes are generally removed after a few days. After a pneumonectomy, the empty chest cavity gradually fills with fluid. Following a lobectomy, the remaining lung and the other structures in the chest shift around and fill the space left behind.

Patients gradually increase their activities after discharge from the hospital. Pain from incisions decreases over time. Most patients return to work within six to eight weeks.

Everyone makes mistakes. For me, smoking was one of them. Once I stopped feeling guilty and angry at myself, I started focusing on living every day that I am blessed with to the fullest.

Catherine, 63
Patient

6

Radiation Therapy

Approximately 60 percent of lung cancer patients undergo radiation therapy. Because cancer cells grow more rapidly than normal cells, they are more susceptible to damage by radiation. These fast-growing cells are particularly vulnerable when they are new and dividing. When radiation damages the structure of the cancer cells, they are unable to duplicate themselves. Normal tissues are also damaged by the radiation but are better able to repair themselves.

Candidates for radiation therapy include patients who cannot benefit from surgery. They also include patients whose cancer has spread to regional lymph nodes or those who aren't strong enough to undergo surgery.

Radiation therapy is also used to alleviate pain caused by lung cancer. For example, radiation may be used to decrease the pain associated with cancer that has spread to bone. It may prevent the cancer from breaking bones, too. Radiation therapy may also be used to shrink a tumor blocking one of the air passages inside the lung, relieving the sensation of shortness of breath.

Types of Radiation Therapy

The first step in radiation therapy is treatment planning. Radiation therapy is administered one of two ways. The most common method is *external beam radiation therapy.* A beam of energy is directed at a tumor from outside the body. The other method is *brachytherapy*, radiation delivered through the nasal passages.

What Happens During Radiation Therapy

A *radiation oncologist* is a doctor who supervises a patient's radiation treatment. He/she has been specially trained in the latest techniques to safely and effectively administer radiation treatment. The radiation oncologists may locate the cancer with the aid of CT scans. With the help of radiation therapy technicians and sometimes a radiation physicist, the oncologist then maps the way the radiation dose will be directed to the cancer. A special shield is custom-made to direct the beam to the precise location. Marks are often made on a patient's skin to help technicians direct the beam correctly. Treatment schedules may vary, but usually last several days to several weeks.

I had thirty radiation treatments. I did become quite fatigued and learned to complete activities in steps, rather than expending a lot of energy at once.

Rosalea, 50
Survivor

The goal of therapy is to apply a higher dose of radiation to the cancerous tumor and a lower dose to normal tissues. The radiation oncologist may use several techniques. He/she can aim the radiation beam at the cancer from different directions, delivering a full dose to the cancer but only a small dose to the normal tissues that the beams must pass through. Or, by dividing the total dose of radiation into smaller doses, the radiation oncologist allows the normal tissues to recover between doses.

During external-beam treatment, the patient is positioned carefully under a machine and the radiation beam is directed to the precise location. The beam may be on for only two to three minutes. The entire process usually takes about fifteen minutes. The patient feels nothing during the treatment, and only hears a soft, whirring sound made by the machine. During the treatment, the technicians will leave the room but will watch and communicate with the patient over an intercom system.

As sick as I was, I did not want the radiation treatments to end. I felt like I was doing something to fight the cancer when I was receiving them. Ending treatments was a difficult part of the recovery process for me.

Lois, 71
Survivor

The second method for the delivery of radiation, brachytherapy, is performed with the help of a pulmonary medicine specialist. Doctors insert a thin plastic tube into a nostril and down into the lung, checking the tube's position with x-rays. Once in place, adjacent to the cancer, the tube is taped to the nose to hold it in position. Radioactive "seeds," which are strung together, are then inserted through the tube and left in place for an hour or two. If additional treatments are required, the plastic tube may be left in place for the next treatment. Sometimes up to four treatments are necessary, performed about one week apart. Many patients have a tendency to cough as the tube passes through the breathing passages. Doctors counter this with cough-suppressing medication.

Side Effects

The effects of radiation therapy on both the cancer and on normal tissues may continue for months after the treatment. Patients should notify their physician if they experience any of the following side effects either during or after radiation therapy.

Fatigue

Fatigue is probably the most common side effect of radiation therapy. Fatigue may set in within hours of receiving treatment or it may not be noticeable for several weeks. Several factors contribute to fatigue. The exposure of normal cells to radiation may cause one to feel tired. The body uses a lot of energy to heal itself during radiation therapy. Coping with the stress of having cancer and daily trips to the treatment center for radiation therapy also drain one's energy.

Cancer specialists recommend that patients decrease their activities and get more rest during this period. They advise patients not to do all the things that they normally do. Asking family members or friends to help with daily chores and obligations is a good idea. Arranging time off from work and working reduced hours are other ways to adapt while undergoing radiation therapy.

Listen until you don't think you can hear anymore about cancer. Read until you can't read anymore about cancer. Talk until people know how you feel and what your needs are.

Carol, 47
Patient

Skin Changes

Radiation therapy does not seriously damage the skin, although some patients experience a sunburn after therapy. Other skin changes are common with radiation treatment. Skin that lies within the path of the radiation beam may become drier, turn pink, and eventually tan slightly. Skin may become less flexible or may even peel. It should be washed very lightly and protected from exposure to the sun. Avoid tight clothing that may rub or irritate affected skin. Do not use lotions or creams to treat skin changes until radiation treatments are completed, unless approved by the staff at the treatment center. Some lotions may coat the skin, decreasing effectiveness of the radiation therapy or interfere with healing.

Dry Mouth and Swallowing Problems

Patients may experience a dry mouth or throat and have difficulty swallowing. Food may stick on occasion. These problems may occur if the esophagus becomes inflamed during radiation therapy. Usually this is a temporary side effect that requires dietary adjustments such as eating soft foods or liquids. Gargling with one-half teaspoon of salt and one-half teaspoon of baking soda mixed in a quart of warm water may help soothe a sore throat.

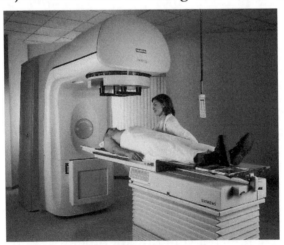

To avoid irritating the esophagus further, specialists recommend that patients avoid tobacco, alcohol or highly carbonated beverages, very hot or cold drinks, "sharp-

A patient receives an external-beam radiation treatment. *Photo courtesy of Siemen's Medical Systems, Inc.*

edged" foods such as pretzels or chips, and spicy foods. To mini-mize swallowing problems, chew food well, cut it into small pieces, or chop or blend. Eat five or six small meals a day. Wear clothing that is loose fitting around the neck.

Hair Loss

Hair loss may occur in the area of treatment. For example, radiation therapy to the head may cause some hair loss from areas of the scalp. Many times, hair grows back after treatments. The amount of hair that grows back depends on the dose of radiation and the type of radiation treatment used. It is important to protect these areas from the sun by wearing a hat, cap, or scarf outdoors. A hairpiece or wig that is needed following cancer treatment is a tax-deductible expense and may be covered by health insurance.

Keep good records of your health and be open and honest about how you are feeling. Don't stay away from a doctor if you are afraid that something is wrong.

Luke, 45
Nurse Practitioner

Dry Cough

The lungs are very sensitive to radiation. An acute form of radiation-induced lung inflammation is called *radiation pneumonitis*. Its most common symptoms are a dry cough, mild fever, and slight shortness of breath on exertion. Doctors treat this with cough suppressants. Radiation pneumonitis occurs during or soon after therapy. Rarely is medication or oxygen required to decrease the inflammation.

A chronic, late-occurring form of lung injury may cause irre-versible lung fibrosis, but this is uncommon. Injury to other impor-tant structures within the body is also uncommon.

New Developments in Radiation Therapy

Several new developments will hopefully increase the effectiveness of radiation on tumors and decrease the impact on normal tissue. It is possible to more accurately deliver radiation to a tumor with computer-assisted methods, or *three-dimensional conformal radiation therapy.* Studies are underway to determine if this is truly advantageous for patients. Protective agents that will increase the resistance of normal tissue to the effects of radiation are also being studied. Finally, in certain situations, radiation therapy combined with chemotherapy is proving more effective than radiation therapy alone.

7

Chemotherapy

Since the early 1990s, tremendous advances have been made in chemotherapy. New drugs and new combinations of drugs have proved more effective against cancer with less severe side effects. Like radiation, chemotherapy damages faster-growing cancer cells.

To determine whether a patient should undergo chemotherapy, health care professionals evaluate one's general health as well as the cancer diagnosis and stage. For example, a person who has not lost much weight and is fairly active might tolerate chemotherapy better than someone who must spend much of the day in bed because of fatigue. Accordingly, before recommending a specific treatment, doctors consider the patient's overall condition, or *performance status*. One of the most commonly used classifications of performance status is the Zubrod scale.

How Chemotherapy Is Given

Chemotherapeutic drugs are usually given (*infused*) directly into a vein (*intravenously*), usually in the forearm. Many of these chemotherapy drugs irritate the small veins in the forearm, so sometimes they are delivered through a thin plastic tube or *catheter* directly into one of the body's large veins such as the *subclavian vein* located under the collar bone. The greater blood flow in the larger vein dilutes the agent before it causes irritation. Sometimes a catheter is attached to a port that is then placed under the skin. Blood samples can be drawn from these implanted catheters so that patients undergo fewer needle sticks during therapy.

Most chemotherapy treatments are given on an outpatient basis in cancer clinics or special areas of the hospitals. It can take up to several hours to receive a treatment. The nurses and doctors, who prepare and administer the potent chemotherapy drugs, are specially trained to do so.

Attitude is everything with chemotherapy. Patients who think they are going to do well, do. Those who think they'll be sick, will be. I've seen this scenario over and over again.

Tory, 33
Nurse

As part of a visit to a chemotherapy clinic, a patient might undergo an exam, blood testing, or x-rays to monitor potential side effects. These test results can also help the staff deliver the proper dose of chemotherapy.

In some instances, patients may need "premedications" to help prevent allergic reactions to the drugs. In other cases, patients may require hydration, with an intravenous fluid, to protect the kidneys.

Side Effects

As with radiation, chemotherapy affects cancer cells because they are dividing more rapidly than most normal cells. However, certain normal cells also grow or divide rapidly and are also affected by the chemotherapy. This accounts for some of the side effects associated with chemotherapy. The bone marrow, where blood cells are made, the digestive system, the reproductive system, and the hair follicles all contain normally fast-growing cells. Most normal cells recover when chemotherapy ends, so many of the side effects will gradually disappear. The length of recovery varies from person to person. Unfortunately, in some instances the side effects may be permanent.

Many patients remember a relative who underwent chemotherapy many years ago and suffered through difficult side effects such as nausea or low blood count. Although current drugs are not free from side effects, in most cases the side effects are less severe. If you're about to receive chemotherapy you may experience some, but not all, of the side effects listed here. Also, be sure to express your concerns about side effects to your physician before undergoing treatment. Be sure to ask:

- What side effects should I expect?
- How long might the side effects last?
- What can I do to cope with the effects?
- When should I seek medical attention for side effects?

Nausea and Vomiting

Chemotherapy may cause nausea and vomiting either by directly affecting the stomach or by affecting the area of the brain that controls vomiting. Sometimes both areas are affected. Not all patients experience nausea. Some patients feel nauseous only

Zubrod Scale
Measurement of Performance Status

Rating	Wellness Level
0	Normal activity, no symptoms
1	Symptomatic, fully ambulatory
2	Symptomatic, in bed less that 50% of time
3	Symptomatic, in bed more than 50% of time
4	100% bedridden

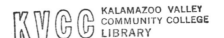

around the time of their treatment. Others feel mildly nauseous all of the time. Doctors may prescribe medicines, *antiemetics,* to counteract the feelings of nausea. Some patients must try different drugs to find the one that works best. The strategies throughout this chapter for coping with side effects are offered by the American Cancer Society. You may wish to try any number of them.

- Eat several small meals during the day to avoid feeling too full.

- Eat and drink slowly. Chew foods well.

- Eat dry foods like toast or crackers when you feel nauseous unless you have mouth sores or a dry mouth.

- Wear loose-fitting clothes.

- Avoid odors that bother you. If the smell of food makes the nausea worse, stay out of the kitchen while food is being cooked.

- Breathe deeply and slowly when you feel nauseous.

- Suck on ice cubes, mints, or tart candies unless you have mouth sores.

There is a lot of apprehension about chemotherapy. People imagine patients being bald, skinny and throwing up. But treatments are so much better than years ago. We are better able to manage the side effects with medication.
Veronica, 48
Radiation Therapist

Hair Loss

Ask your physician if hair loss is likely during chemotherapy. Hair usually grows back once the treatments are over. Sometimes it may grow back in a different color or texture. Hair loss can occur on all parts of the body. The following tips are recommended for hair and scalp during chemotherapy:

- Use mild shampoos.
- Use a soft hair brush.
- Use low heat on your hair dryer.
- Don't use brush rollers to set your hair.
- Don't dye your hair or get a permanent.
- Have your hair cut short, a shorter style will make your hair look thicker and fuller
- Protect your scalp from the sun with a hat, scarf, or sunscreen.

Some people choose to cover their heads with a hat, scarf or wig. To better match your natural color and style, select a wig before much hair loss. Local cancer societies may help you locate a shop or service that provide wigs. If used during cancer therapy, wigs are tax-deductible expenses. Some insurance policies cover the cost as well, if the wigs are prescribed by a physician. There are also wig "banks" that let people borrow hairpieces or wigs.

We used to have patients stay over night in the hospital for chemo. Now we have some people coming in during their lunch hour. People go about their daily routines, and chemotherapy is part of that.

Brian, 36
Radiation Therapist

Fatigue

Fatigue is a common symptom among patients undergoing chemotherapy. Patients may notice an improvement in energy levels once treatment is over. Sometimes, for a number of different reasons, some level of fatigue persists.

Physicians can help by watching for medically treatable causes of fatigue, such as a low red blood cell count (*anemia*). Red blood cells carry oxygen throughout the body and provide energy. Anemia may also cause shortness of breath, a fast heart rate, and dizziness. Anemia may be treated with either a blood transfusion or medication that helps the body make more red blood cells. To reduce fatigue, specialists further recommend that you:

- Limit your activities. Do only those things that are most important to you.
- Take several short naps or breaks during the day.
- Some people find that taking short walks or exercising lightly helps decrease fatigue.
- Maintain good nutrition. Try to eat a well balanced diet.
- Ask for help when you need it.

Patients often find that they need to make lifestyle changes to cope with lower energy levels. Talking to the doctor, staff, family and friends about the frustration of being fatigued can also be very helpful.

Infection

Patients receiving chemotherapy are likely to get infections. Chemotherapy affects the bone marrow, the tissue that makes white blood cells. White blood cells fight many types of infections. Physicians check the white blood cell count frequently during chemotherapy. A medication, called *granulocyte colony stimulating factor (G-CSF)*, which stimulates the body's production of white blood cells may be given to prevent the white blood cell count from falling too far below normal. If the white blood cell count drops too far despite treatment with G-CSF, chemotherapy may be postponed or the dose of chemotherapy decreased. To avoid infection:

- Stay away from people who have diseases that you can catch, such as a cold, the flu, measles or chicken pox.
- Wash your hands often during the day, especially after using the bathroom.
- Clean your rectal area gently but thoroughly after each bowel movement. Notify your doctor or nurse if this area becomes irritated or if you have hemorrhoids.
- Stay away from children who have recently received vaccinations.
- Clean cuts and scrapes right away.
- Wear gloves when gardening or cleaning up after pets or small children.
- Use a soft toothbrush that won't hurt your gums.
- Be careful not to cut or nick yourself.

Be alert for these signs of infection:

- Fever over 100ºF
- Chills
- Sweating
- A burning feeling when you urinate
- A severe cough or sore throat
- Unusual vaginal discharge or itching

I believe it was the strength of our love that enabled my husband to win his battle with lung cancer. We celebrated life together for 10 years after his recovery. We bought a motor home and traveled throughout the country.

Shirley, 64
Wife of Survivor

- Redness, swelling, or tenderness, especially around an incision, wound, sore, pimple, or site of an intravenous catheter

Report any signs of infection to your doctor right away. This is especially important if your white blood cell count is low. If you have a fever, don't use aspirin or acetaminophen without your doctor's approval.

Blood Clotting Problems

Chemotherapy may affect the body's ability to make *platelets*, blood cells that help form clots. Like white blood cells, platelets are made by the bone marrow. Patients with a low platelet count tend to bleed or bruise more easily from minor injuries, cuts, or abrasions. Bleeding may also occur in the urine, coloring it red or pink or into the stomach and intestines, coloring the stool red or black. Alert your physician if you notice any of these symptoms. Your doctor may monitor your platelet count while you are receiving chemotherapy. If the platelet count drops too low, he/she may order a transfusion of platelets. To further avoid clotting problems:

- Don't take medication without first checking with your doctor. This includes aspirin and aspirin-free pain relievers like acetaminophen and ibuprofen. These drugs decrease platelet function. Many over-the-counter medicines contain aspirin, so read labels carefully.
- Don't drink alcoholic beverages unless your doctor says it's okay.
- Use a soft toothbrush to clean your teeth.
- Take care not to nick yourself when using scissors, needles, knives, or tools.

- Clean your nose by gently blowing into a soft tissue.
- Be careful not to burn yourself while cooking.
- Avoid activities that may cause injury.

Mouth, Gum and Throat Problems

Chemotherapy may cause sores in the mouth and throat. It may also dry or irritate tissues in the mouth or cause them to bleed. Mouth sores can also become infected. Good oral care is important. The following may help keep your mouth, throat and gums healthy:

- If possible, see your dentist before chemotherapy to have your teeth cleaned and cavities filled.
- Brush and floss your teeth properly, using a soft toothbrush. Hard bristles may damage tissues.
- Rinse your toothbrush well after use and store it in a dry place.
- Avoid commercial mouthwashes that contain a lot of salt or alcohol. Ask your doctor or nurse to recommend a mouthwash. Your dentist may also recommend a fluoride rinse or special gel for oral care.

> *Everyone has a perception of cancer based on past experiences. Keep in mind that each case is different and focus on your own.*
>
> *Holly, 45*
> *Social Worker*

Notify your doctor if sores develop in your mouth. If sores make eating difficult, you may wish to:

- Ask your doctor for medication to make the sores less painful.
- Eat foods cold or at room temperature since hot foods may irritate a tender mouth.

- Choose soft foods to eat such as ice cream, milkshakes, baby food, bananas, applesauce, mashed potatoes, cooked cereals, soft-boiled or scrambled eggs, cottage cheese, custards, and puddings.
- Avoid acidic foods such as tomatoes, spicy or salty foods, or rough or coarse foods.

If mouth dryness occurs, try the following:

- Drink plenty of liquids.

- Suck on ice chips, popsicles, or sugarless hard candy.
- Moisten foods with butter, margarine, gravy or broth.
- Dunk crisp, dry foods in mild liquids.
- Eat soft foods.
- Use lip balm for dry lips.

Keeping a journal can be helpful for tracking information, symptoms, and medications, but it can also help you sort out emotions. Write about your frustrations and fears, but focus on constructive thoughts.

Rebecca, 40
Social Worker

Diarrhea

Chemotherapeutic drugs may affect the cells that line the intestine, producing loose or watery stools. Notify your physician if diarrhea lasts for more than twenty-four hours or is associated with abdominal pain or cramping. Also contact your physician before taking any over-the-counter antidiarrheal medicine. Intravenous fluids are sometimes necessary if diarrhea becomes severe. If diarrhea becomes a problem:

- Eat smaller amounts of food, but eat more often.

- Avoid high fiber foods that may make diarrhea worse (raw vegetables, whole grains, beans, seeds, popcorn).
- Avoid coffee, tea, alcohol and sweets. Also avoid fried, greasy or highly spiced foods.
- Drink plenty of fluids to replace those you have lost through diarrhea.

Nerve and Muscle Problems

Certain chemotherapeutic drugs affect the nerves throughout the body. One common effect is *peripheral neuropathy,* usually tingling, burning, weakness, or numbness in the hands and/or feet. Other symptoms that are nerve related include loss of balance, clumsiness, difficulty picking up objects and buttoning clothing, walking problems, jaw pain, hearing loss, stomach pain, and constipation. Some drugs affect the muscles directly, making them sore, weak, or tired. If you experience nerve or muscle problems:

- Carefully pick up hot or sharp objects if you have noted clumsiness.
- Carefully step in and out of the tub or shower to avoid falls.
- Do not wear slippery shoes.

Changes in the Skin and Nails

Chemotherapy may cause minor skin problems and changes in the nails. Skin may dry out, redden, itch, peel, or develop acne. Fingernails and toenails may darken, become cracked, or develop vertical lines. Certain cancer drugs darken the veins in the skin where they are infused. These darkened areas usually fade over several months, after the treatments stop.

Some areas of previously radiated skin may develop "radiation recall" during chemotherapy. During or shortly after treatment, the skin may again turn red and itch or burn. These reactions should be reported to a physician or nurse. The following guidelines may be helpful if you have problems with skin and nails:

- It is okay to use nail strengthening remedies sold over the counter.
- Wear gloves when doing dishes, and working in the garden or around the house.
- Check with your doctor or nurse about using a sunscreen. Wear long-sleeved shirts, pants, and hats.

Most skin problems are not serious. However, certain chemotherapy agents can injure the skin and surrounding tissue if they leak out of the vein during an infusion. Tell your doctor or nurse right away if you feel any burning or pain when receiving drugs through an IV. Allergic reactions to chemotherapy drugs often involve the skin. Notify the doctor or nurse if you develop severe itching, hives, or a rash, or if you begin wheezing or have trouble breathing.

Kidney and Bladder Problems

Some chemotherapeutic drugs irritate the bladder or can damage the kidneys. In general, drinking plenty of fluids will help. Your physicians will indicate which drugs may cause problems. Some anticancer drugs cause the urine to change color (to orange, red, or yellow) or to take on a strong medicine-like odor. Notify your doctor or nurse if you notice:

- Pain or burning when you urinate
- Frequent urination

- A feeling that you must urinate right away
- Reddish or brown urine
- Fever
- Chills

Sexual Problems

Chemotherapy may affect the sexual organs and sexual functioning in both men and women. In men, anticancer drugs may reduce the sperm count or reduce sperm movement, leading to a decrease in fertility. This may be temporary or permanent. If fertility is an issue for you, discuss it with your doctor before treatment. Some patients may want to consider banking sperm, freezing it for later use.

In women, anticancer drugs may reduce hormonal output, producing irregular periods or no periods during treatment. One might experience menopause-like symptoms such as hot flashes, itching, burning, or dry vaginal tissues. Using a water-soluble vaginal lubricant may help. Also, decreased vaginal lubrication during treatment may increase the risk of infection. Wearing cotton underwear that can "breathe" and pantyhose with a cotton lining may help. Temporary or permanent infertility can also occur in women. Pregnancy is not advisable during treatment since anticancer drugs may cause birth defects.

Sexual feelings vary widely during chemotherapy. Some people feel closer than ever to their partners and note enhanced sexual interest. Others find that the physical and emotional stress interferes with sexual desire. Some partners may worry that physical intimacy may harm the person who has cancer. Sometimes, partners mistakenly fear that they will "catch" the cancer through intimate contact.

Talking about feelings is important and helpful. Many people discover that physical intimacy takes on a new meaning and character. Hugging, touching, holding, and cuddling may become more important while sexual intercourse may become less important. It is up to you and your partner to determine together what is pleasurable and satisfying.

8

Multimodality Therapy

Previously, we examined the main methods physicians use to treat patients with lung cancer—surgery, radiation therapy, and chemotherapy. In this chapter, we'll explore the benefits of treating patients with *multimodality therapy,* a combination of treatments. It may be the most promising advance in lung cancer treatment in twenty years, especially for patients with early-stage disease. The multimodality approach involves a team of doctors administering more than one form of treatment. For example, a patient may undergo chemotherapy followed by surgery, or receive a combination of radiation and chemotherapy.

Unfortunately, one-half to three-fourths of all lung cancer patients are never referred to oncologists for multimodality treatment. Why would so many doctors and patients not take advantage of new, improved treatments? There are several reasons.

Why Multimodality Therapy Is Under-Used

In many cases, patients are simply unaware of the state-of-the-art treatments offered through clinical trials. In other instances, chemotherapy still has a bad reputation. Patients sometimes are not aware of advances of chemotherapy and are reluctant to participate in a clinical trial if it means undergoing chemotherapy. Many patients mistakenly think that participating in a clinical trial makes them part of an unreliable experiment. Clinical trials offer a chance to receive some of the newest treatments available—treatments that have undergone rigorous scientific study and show promise. Other times, clinical trials may be far from home or are otherwise impractical. More on clinical trials in the next chapter.

Side effects can be worse when chemotherapy and radiation are administered concurrently. Irritation of the esophageal lining can make it very difficult for patients to eat. Be hopeful! Response and cure rates are higher with this method.

David, 53
Radiation Therapist

Doctors and other health-care professionals may also be unaware of new treatments. Those who are aware may doubt whether the new approaches are better. At the same time, physicians may question whether their patients are suitable for a particular clinical trial. Enrolling patients in a clinical trial takes additional time and effort, and there may be few incentives.

Unfortunately, many doctors have a pessimistic view of lung cancer treatment. They may view lung cancer as an incurable disease and act as if it were untreatable. In many instances lung cancer does prove to be incurable. Still, this does not mean that treatment would not improve the length and quality of a patient's life. Nevertheless, some doctors are reluctant to recommend any treatment that may have side effects if it would not prolong life significantly.

Multimodality therapy also requires close coordination among medical specialists. This may be difficult to coordinate in many practice settings.

How Multimodality Therapy Is Best Delivered

Multimodality therapy is best administered by a team of physicians who confer regularly on a case. However, many health-care professionals practice a medical specialty-oriented approach when it comes to caring for patients with lung cancer. That means patients are referred to a series of specialists, but the specialists do not work as a team. For example, a patient may be referred to a surgeon for surgery. Next, the patient may be sent to a radiation oncologist to receive appropriate radiation therapy. Both specialists use their skills to treat the lung cancer patient. However, they may give little or no thought to coordinating treatment plans, or to enrolling the patient in a clinical trial of state-of-the-art, multimodality therapy.

My doctors worked as a team and discussed my case. I was told what they concluded. I felt so informed. It was wonderful. I survived adenocarcinoma.

Rosalea, 50
Survivor

Consider the example of Mrs. Jones, who is sent from doctor to doctor. Let's say Mrs. Jones is generally in good health, but a routine chest x-ray shows a lung mass or tumor. Her family doctor refers her to a pulmonary physician for further evaluation. Eight days later, when she meets with the pulmonary specialist, he notes that the mass is located near Mrs. Jones' chest wall, far from the center of her chest. It may be hard for the pulmonary specialist to biopsy the mass and to determine if it is a cancer by using a bronchoscope to look inside the breathing passages. So, Mrs. Jones is referred to another specialist, an interventional radiologist, who will perform a needle biopsy of the nodule to determine if it is a cancer.

This approach to treatment occurs every day. Medically, Mrs. Jones would *not* be harmed by waiting two or three weeks for her diagnosis. A cancer would not grow much in that period of time. It is, however, inconvenient and stressful for a patient to wait so long for an answer.

A multidisciplinary approach would not only simplify the process for Mrs. Jones but would also allow her to receive optimal treatment. All the health-care professionals who might ordinarily care for a patient with lung cancer would take part in all the steps: diagnosis, staging, therapy, even long-term follow-up.

> *I was told I couldn't have chemo, surgery or radiation because of my poor lung condition. One doctor believed I could have surgery. Another believed I could have radiation. I had them both and I am still here.*
>
> *Michelle, 38*
> *Survivor*

What if the family doctor could confer with *both* the pulmonary specialist and the interventional radiologist when he/she first gets Mrs. Jones' chest x-ray report? All the doctors might realize that a needle biopsy is the best method to examine the mass seen on Mrs. Jones' chest x-ray. The family doctor might refer Mrs. Jones directly for a needle biopsy, saving her an unnecessary trip to the pulmonary specialist and probably many days of worry.

Whether the health-care professionals sit together face-to-face in a weekly multidisciplinary conference or confer closely in other ways, the goal of multimodality therapy is the same: to involve all specialists from the beginning and to provide state-of-the-art consultation and treatment for the patient.

9

Treatment for Stages of Cancer

Today, lung cancer can be treated. The medical advances described in the previous chapters make a significant difference in treating lung cancer, both in quality of life and in survival. However, negative attitudes about prognosis among both patients and doctors must change if more patients are to be helped. Experts estimate that up to 70 percent of lung cancer patients are not receiving the best possible treatment. Why? They aren't being referred to cancer specialists.

When making treatment recommendations for patients with lung cancer, doctors consider a range of factors. Age is an important factor, as is overall medical condition. Patients who are frail are generally less able to undergo combination therapies. On the other hand, patients who are active and able to perform strenuous activities are more likely to get good results from multimodality therapy. Other factors, such as the extent of any spread of the cancer, also influence the type of treatment. For example, surgical removal of a tumor is generally not an option for those whose cancer has spread beyond the lung, into the nearby lymph nodes.

Finally, doctors consider the generally recommended treatments for each stage of non-small cell and small cell lung cancer.

Treatment Options for Small Cell Lung Cancer

Limited Stage Small Cell Lung Cancer
- Chemotherapy with radiation therapy
  This combination therapy is used to control both distant and local cancer within the chest. *Prophylactic cranial irradiation* (PCI) may be used to decrease the likelihood that cancer will recur in the brain.
- Chemotherapy with possible PCI
- Chemotherapy and surgery with possible PCI
  Patients found to have very early small cell lung cancer may be successfully treated with surgical resection to remove local tumor, followed by chemotherapy to prevent any distant metastases.

Extensive Stage Small Cell Lung Cancer
- Chemotherapy with possible PCI
  Chemotherapy is used to treat the cancer with or without PCI to decrease the likelihood that cancer will recur in the brain.
- Radiation
  Radiation therapy aims to treat symptoms produced by distant metastases.

Treatment Options for Non-Small Cell Lung Cancer

Stage IA

- Surgery alone
  This is the main treatment for the earliest stage of non-small lung cancer.
- Radiation therapy alone
  This is given to patients who refuse surgery or are not strong enough for surgery.

Stage IB

- Chemotherapy and surgery in clinical trials
  Generally, patients with larger cancers that have not spread to the lymph nodes face a high risk of cancer recurrence elsewhere in the body after surgery. Therefore, specialists now consider chemotherapy either before or after surgery to be optimal treatment. This additional treatment is known as adjuvant therapy, or neoadjuvant therapy.
- Surgery alone
- Surgery and radiation therapy

There are still some people out there that hear the word cancer and are sure that they are going to die. We've advanced in cancer treatment. By giving up, you could really be shortchanging yourself.

Patrick, 34
Pulmonary
Rehabilitation Specialist

Stage IIA and IIB

- Chemotherapy and surgery in clinical trials
  Patients with cancers, small or large, that have spread to lymph nodes inside the lungs also face a high risk of

cancer developing elsewhere in the body after surgery. Optimal therapy for these patients includes chemotherapy either before or after surgery.

- Surgery alone
  Recent studies suggest that routine postoperative radiation therapy in these patients may actually decrease survival.

Stage IIIA

- Chemotherapy and radiation therapy
  Studies have proved that a combination of chemotherapy and radiation therapy is better than radiation therapy alone for treating patients with stage IIIA disease in otherwise generally good health. Radiation therapy aims to control the cancer in the chest, while chemotherapy seeks to destroy any cancer cells that have spread elsewhere in the body.
- Chemotherapy and surgery with possible radiation therapy
  Clinical trials are underway to determine if surgery is better than radiation therapy at controlling the part of the cancer inside the chest, while chemotherapy attacks any cancer cells that have spread elsewhere in the body. Other clinical trials are designed to find out if surgery followed by chemotherapy and radiation therapy improves survival.
- Radiation therapy alone
  This was standard treatment for many years. It remains standard treatment for patients with poor performance status.

- Surgery and radiation therapy
- Surgery alone
  Not recommended, except for a select few patients.

Stage IIIB

- Chemotherapy and radiation therapy
  A combination of chemotherapy and radiation therapy
  has long been standard for patients with stage IIIB
  non-small cell lung cancer. Patients
  must have a good performance status.
  Radiation therapy aims to control the
  local cancer in the chest, while
  chemotherapy seeks to destroy any
  cancer cells that have spread
  elsewhere.
- Radiation therapy alone
  This is commonly given to stage IIIB
  patients who do not have good
  performance status.
- Other treatments followed by surgery
  Surgery has not been shown to
  improve survival unless used in
  combination with other therapies.
  Patients must have good performance
  status. Such multimodality therapy is
  usually given as part of a clinical trial.
- Chemotherapy alone

After my dad finished his chemotherapy treatments, we decorated his room with streamers and balloons, brought in a cake, and invited family and his health care team. Plan something positive for when treatments are finished.

Catlin, 16
Daughter of Survivor

Stage IV

- Chemotherapy
  Chemotherapy has been shown to lengthen life and improve quality of life for patients with advanced lung cancer who have good performance status. Using chemotherapy with the best supportive care may be thought of as multimodality therapy.

- Radiation therapy alone
  Often used to treat symptoms from distant metastases, such as pain from a metastasis to bone.

- Best supportive care
  This is given to improve a patient's function and comfort as much as possible. It is not aimed at killing or shrinking the cancer. It is for patients with advanced disease and poor performance status. Best supportive care may be combined with other treatments.

- Local or internal radiation therapy
  This treatment may open air passages blocked by cancer, relieving shortness of breath or clearing up infections.

Non-Small Cell Treatment
Conventional vs. State of the Art

Stage	Conventional	State of the Art
IA	Surgery alone or Radiation alone	Surgery alone
IB	Surgery alone or Radiation alone	Surgery & Chemotherapy
IIA/B	Surgery & Radiation or Radiation alone	Surgery, Chemotherapy and possible Radiation

IIIA	Surgery & Radiation	Surgery, Chemotherapy and possible Radiation
IIIB	Chemotherapy & Radiation	Chemotherapy & Radiation
IV	Best Supportive Care Chemotherapy	Chemotherapy Best Supportive Care

Identifying Optimal Lung Cancer Treatment

- Be an informed consumer.
- Seek treatment from a cancer specialist.
- Find out if your doctor, hospital, clinic, or group of doctors has a multidisciplinary clinic devoted to treating patients with lung cancer.
- Make sure that you know the stage of your lung cancer. Ask your doctor for the TNM classification. Make sure that you understand what it means and how it was determined.
- Find out if you need mediastinoscopy to evaluate the lymph nodes in the center of your chest. If your doctors don't think it is necessary, ask them to explain why.
- Find out if your doctor or hospital has clinical trials available for your type and stage of lung cancer. If they don't, ask them to find a place that does.

My wife gave me no choice. I had to stay involved in daily activities. She pushed me right through the treatments and helped me to succeed. Having a motivator makes a huge difference.

R.J., 52
Survivor

Seeking Help

The treatment recommendations outlined in this chapter reflect current options generally prescribed for the different types and stages of lung cancer. New developments may change these recommendations. Knowing important facts, such as the stage of your disease will help you discover the very latest treatment recommendations. You should also find out if any new clinical trials are available. The Cancer Information Service provides such information. Call 1-800-4-CANCER (1-800-422-6237), or TTY at 1-800-332-8615. This number will connect you with a trained information specialist who can answer your questions. The National Cancer Institute has several booklets available that can be sent to you upon request. Their address is listed in the Resources section of this book. For those with Internet access, the National Cancer Institute has an extensive web site for health-care professionals and the public called CancerNet at http://cancernet.nci.cih.gov. From this web site, one may access a database called PDQ, which provides updates on cancer and cancer treatments.

Don't ever say you 'can't.' Someone out there has been cured of every kind of cancer. If they can do it, you can do it.

Susan, 42
Nurse Practitioner

10

Clinical Trials

Should you participate in a clinical trial? You may not know enough about them to make an informed decision. In order to consider a clinical trial as a treatment option, it is important to understand how they work.

A clinical trial is a research study conducted with patients. In the field of cancer research, the goal of such a trial is often to compare a new treatment to a standard treatment. A clinical trial may also test methods of preventing cancer. It is important to remember that participants in clinical trials do not receive untested treatments—they are not "guinea pigs." New treatments are offered to patients in clinical trials only after extensive laboratory research has demonstrated that they are at least as good as, and potentially much better than, standard therapies.

The knowledge gained from clinical trials accounts for much of the progress that has been made in treating patients with cancer. Many of today's best standard treatments were first available to patients in clinical trials.

How Clinical Trials Work

Once researchers identify a promising new treatment, doctors and researchers write a treatment plan, called a *protocol,* for a clinical trial. The new treatment plan might involve a new anticancer drug, a combination of treatment methods, or new methods for cancer prevention. Before a clinical trial can be offered to patients, an institutional review board (IRB) must approve the protocol for an organization—cancer center, hospital, clinic, or medical school—where the trial will be conducted.

Many people are enthused about participating in clinical trials because they offer more innovative and advanced treatment options. Every treatment poses risks. Consider the merits of the protocol and the advantages.
James, 61
Oncologist

The review board includes doctors, researchers, and members of the public. The board follows strict ethical guidelines for the conduct of medical research supported by both the federal government and the international community. The Food and Drug Administration (FDA) and the Office of Protection from Research Risks (OPRR) periodically review the conduct of the review board. The board periodically monitors the results of the clinical trial to make sure that ethical practices are followed.

Participating in a Clinical Trial

Participation in a clinical trial is strictly voluntary. You may stop participating in a clinical trial at any time before, during, or after you have received the new treatment. Upon leaving the trial, if any medical problems result from the trial treatment, you will continue to receive appropriate medical care.

How do you enroll in a trial? Ask your doctor or oncologist to help you find a trial that is suitable. He/she will ask you to sign a consent form after reviewing all the details of the clinical trial with you, including the potential benefits and risks.

Clinical trials are offered in hospitals, cancer centers, doctor's offices, and clinics throughout the United States and internationally. However, some trials are available only at certain locations. Clinical trials are sponsored by a number of different organizations, both public and private. The National Cancer Institute sponsors many clinical trials. It works through a number of other organizations, including its own designated cancer centers, the Cooperative Group Clinical Trials Program, and the Community Clinical Oncology Program (CCOP). The CCOP helps community physicians take part in clinical trials. The National Cancer Institute also has an agreement with the Department of Veterans Affairs to allow eligible patients to participate in clinical trials. Pharmaceutical companies also sponsor clinical trials. Additional information is available from the Resource section in the back of this book.

I was fearful of the tests and treatments that I would encounter. But when you realize that having surgery or chemotherapy is your only chance of surviving, it helps you do almost anything.

Richard, 65
Patient

Phases of a Clinical Trial

You may hear a clinical trial described as a phase I or phase III trial. Clinical trials are typically divided into four phases.

Phase I Clinical Trial

A phase I clinical trial determines the safest dose or best method to use when giving a new treatment. Since this may be the first time that the new treatment has been given to people, careful attention is paid to any side effects that may develop. Patients asked to enroll in this type of trial are unlikely to benefit from standard treatments.

Phase II Clinical Trial

Once the safe dosage or method of administration has been determined in phase I, a phase II trial is organized to determine if the treatment is effective in decreasing the size of a tumor. The number of patients responding favorably is also noted. Health-care professionals and patients hope to see a high response rate in the group enrolled in the trial.

Phase III Clinical Trial

Usually, only those treatments that have shown to have strong positive effects and acceptable side effects in phases I and II are tested in a phase III trial. If several new trial treatments are available, patients will be randomly assigned to one. A phase III clinical trial then compares the effects of the new treatment with those of a standard treatment. To determine which treatment is the best, large numbers of participants may be required for a phase III trial.

Phase IV Clinical Trial

The monitoring and data collection that is required after a treatment is first approved for use by the FDA is sometimes described as phase IV of clinical testing.

A clinical trial ends when the number of patients needed to obtain valid results have completed their assigned treatment. Some trials end sooner if the new treatment proves to be clearly more effective than the standard treatment. If the new treatment proves less effective than the standard treatment, the trial may also stop early.

Advantages of Clinical Trials

- Participants receive therapy that is likely to produce better results than standard treatments.
- Patients are among the first to receive new therapy.
- Responses to treatments, including side effects, are carefully monitored by doctors who specialize in cancer treatment.
- Patients contribute to the development of new treatments that may help others.

Disadvantages of Clinical Trials

- New therapies may not prove more effective than standard treatments.
- Side effects of a new treatment may be unexpected or more severe than expected.
- Some costs of the treatments given during the clinical trial may not be covered by your insurance company.
- Patients may have to travel a long distance to a specialized center to participate in a trial since the new treatment may not be available everywhere.

Questions to Ask Before Participating in a Clinical Trial

How does the new treatment that I might receive in the clinical trial differ from the standard treatment for my condition? This is an important question. You should have some idea of the rationale behind the new treatment—why doctors and researchers think it might be better.

Who may participate in the clinical trial? What are the eligibility criteria? How is that determined? Remember that being turned down for a study does not mean that you cannot get better, it simply means that you aren't the type of patient that the trial was designed for.

> *I really appreciate it when people offer their assistance and support before I have to ask for help. I feel like I'm a burden on others, but it is important to ask for help when you need it.*
>
> *Phil, 85*
> *Patient*

What are the potential risks if I agree to participate? How will the treatment affect me physically or affect my day-to-day life? Answers to these questions are usually spelled out in the informed consent form that you must sign before participating. Be sure that you understand what the form says. If you don't understand it at first, don't be afraid to ask someone to explain it to you.

How long will the proposed treatment take? How many weeks or months? How many visits per week? Will I have to travel to another facility or another city for any part of the treatment? Be realistic regarding your willingness to make the commitment required to participate in a trial.

Will the cost of any treatments or special tests required by the clinical trial be covered by my insurance? If the trial is sponsored by a drug company, will the sponsor cover the additional cost? Your insurance plan may not cover all the costs because it may consider trials to be experimental therapy.

11

Coping Emotionally

Anytime a diagnosis of cancer is made, patients are usually flooded with such feelings as fear, anger, or anxiety. These are all understandable human emotions. But, following a diagnosis of lung cancer, many patients are forced to deal with painful emotions, unlike those faced by other cancer patients. There is often a stigma attached to lung cancer—the underlying belief that a patient, because he/she smoked, is responsible for the disease. Consequently, the patient may experience feelings of isolation and abandonment. Friends and relatives may be angry and may blame the patient for getting lung cancer. It is important for family and friends to acknowledge this attitude, however subtle it may be. A loved one needs care and support from them.

Smoker's Guilt

Smokers are often angry at themselves, too. In addition to blaming themselves for getting cancer, they may feel guilty for having caused emotional pain for loved ones. Their guilt may also arise from concern over expenses and inconveniences to others.

There is often a general feeling of having done wrong, of feeling hopeless and helpless. Smokers experiencing such guilt should remember:

- Nicotine addiction is powerful. It's difficult for many to quit smoking. This does not mean you are a weak person.
- You had no intentions of bringing disease upon yourself when you started smoking.
- Smoking was an easy habit to start. You may have started out of peer pressure. Perhaps you wanted to fit in, to belong to a circle of friends.
- There may be other reasons why you smoked. Perhaps it was a way of relaxing, coping with anxiety. Maybe it increased your alertness, helped you feel better, or cope better.
- Cancer may strike anyone. No one asks for it.
- Don't forget that support is available for dealing with these feelings. Don't fall into the isolation trap—it has a way of amplifying negative emotions.

> *I really wanted someone to talk to, but I didn't feel comfortable going to a support group with a room full of strangers. I called ALCASE, a national support organization, at 1-800-298-2436. I was paired with a phone buddy. She has been very informative and supportive.*
>
> *Mary Lou, 79*
> *Patient*

Stop believing that you caused your disease. Now is the time to lighten your load of self-doubt, self-criticism, and guilt for whatever you feel you have done wrong. Forgive yourself for any sense of wrongdoing, just as you might have forgiven others at times in your life.

Stress Management

Few things are more stressful than a diagnosis of cancer. Reducing stress has a powerful influence on the body and the course of a disease. Increasing numbers of studies on the mind/body relationship demonstrate the connections between our thoughts, feelings, attitudes, and beliefs as they affect our behaviors, immune system, and overall physiology. A strong immune system, of course, is necessary to resist infection, illness, and disease. Chronic psychological stress seems to be *immunosuppressive*, meaning it hampers the immune system's ability to function optimally. It has been shown that stressful life events—particularly negative changes like divorce, bereavement, and other major losses—can increase the risk of developing diseases of any kind.

Being connected to others who are going through the same thing is really a source of strength for me. I have developed relationships with other patients and we check up on each other. Cultivate camaraderie and cherish it.

Mary Alice, 64
Patient

Research continues on the relationship between stress and cancer. Studies with animals have shown that chronic stress impairs the ability of cells to repair structural damage, which is believed to influence the onset of cancer. When we experience significant stress we become susceptible to the damaging effects of *cortisol*, a stress hormone that in excessive amounts may weaken the immune system. Stress has varying effects on individuals according to their personality, coping skills, life circumstances, and the availability of social support. Developing effective stress-management skills is particularly important for someone with cancer, who requires a strong immune system. Stress-management skills may be learned and developed with practice.

Eliminate Stressors

Stress management begins by first assessing your stress level. Review the major negative stress factors in your life and eliminate as many as you can. In this way you can free up more of your energy to deal effectively with what is most important now. Ask yourself what matters most in life. Put yourself at the top of your priority list. A certain amount of self-centeredness is required for optimal self-care. Practice saying "yes" to yourself and "no" to others when it is better to do so. Identify things that drain your energy and eliminate as many as possible. Replace them with the things that fill you up, those people and activities that enliven you. Remember what is fun and what makes you laugh. These necessary additions will help balance the more serious aspects of life with an illness.

Lung cancer is not talked about enough. Maybe if more people speak up we will get more help and understanding.

Helen, 50
Survivor

Nutrition, Sleep, and Exercise

Stress management includes a nutritious diet that is low in sugar, caffeine, and processed foods. Good nutrition provides the nutrients that help to repair the body. Adequate sleep and rest cannot be underestimated in helping to cope better. Adequate exercise may release toxic stress hormones stored in the body and stimulate *endorphins*, or "feel-good" hormones. Discuss any physical limitations of exercise with your doctor. Relaxation audiotapes may be useful in stress management. Basic, deep abdominal breathing is very effective at reducing anxiety. A simple but effective exercise is to close your eyes and take a deep breath, seeing yourself filled with vitality and peace and healing. As you exhale, imagine that you are also releasing any tension or negative feelings.

Touch

Touch is a remarkable stress reducer. Allow for as many hugs in a day as you can. It's okay to ask for a hug or even initiate one yourself. Cuddling a pet works too. Body massages can be very soothing, both physically and emotionally.

Expressing Emotions

Patients often ask whether emotions or personality have anything to do with developing cancer. A positive attitude is certainly helpful but does not guarantee an extended life. Suppressing our feelings, however, produces significant stress. Covering up and burying genuine feelings like fear and sadness by putting on a happy face for others may prove harmful. Of course, certain emotions are distressing. Yet our feelings can serve as messengers, signaling needed reevaluation or correction. They can help us make the best choices. If we are reluctant to openly express them, the body often does the communicating for us in symptoms or illness. Feelings are not right or wrong—they are human.

Learning new ways to express feelings may be especially helpful for smokers. For some, smoking is a temporary fix for difficult or uncomfortable feelings like anger, worry, loneliness, or fear. The smoking habit may keep one from learning other more appropriate ways to experience and resolve situations that evoke strong emotional responses. Lung cancer patients often withdraw and suffer alone which can intensify those feelings and hamper healing.

Social Support

Social support during a life crisis helps reduce stress. Many support groups are available for people with cancer and their loved ones. Simply being with people who are living with cancer, people who can relate to your experiences and your feelings, can be enormously helpful. Support groups allow people to discuss a variety of issues related to having cancer. They usually focus on daily living, relationship, and communication problems and provide a place to discuss subjects or feelings you are uncomfortable sharing with family members. It can help to hear how others are coping with cancer.

My mother was strong in her faith. It really helped her to get cards from church members and know that others were praying for her. She believes that this is why she survived and pulled through.

Melanie, 24
Daughter of Survivor

Numerous studies have shown that people with social support have lower mortality from a variety of diseases than those without. Cancer patients with stronger social support may actually live longer than patients with weaker social support. It is positively associated with both better adjustment and longer survival. A ten-year study of women with metastatic breast cancer revealed the positive effects of psychological and social support on their survival. The women who participated in a weekly support group experienced fewer mood swings, less phobia and pain, and survived twice as long as those who were not in a support group. This therapy focused on expressing fears, anger, anxiety, and depression. The women were also encouraged to be assertive and grieve for their losses. Similar studies have demonstrated the benefits of social support on longer survival for people with melanoma and lymphoma.

How strong is your social support system? How connected do you feel to other people? You may have chosen a life of relative isolation to feel safe. But it can also be painfully lonely, especially during a life crisis like major illness. We all need others. We are interdependent. It is okay to reach out, even though it may at first feel awkward. You may want to think about the important people in your life. Who accepts you for who you are? Who do you trust completely? Who shows an interest in your well-being? Who has coped with similar problems? Who could help you with daily activities? Who could be there for you if you opened up more and nurtured that relationship? Serving the needs of others and reciprocating good deeds are gifts for the givers, too.

Counseling

Counseling takes many forms. It includes individual psychotherapy, group therapy, support groups, and family therapy. Counseling may prove most beneficial for those who suspect they have powerful buried feelings that are hampering the body's freedom to heal. It is possible to overcome feelings of self-blame, anger, anxiety, and depression with renewed well-being. People who have a positive sense of self-worth tend to take better care of themselves.

Individual counseling may help you evaluate the changes you need to make to improve the quality of your life. It may assist you too in expressing your feelings and needs with others, improving relationship dynamics, and becoming more assertive as needed with medical providers and others.

Family counseling may be helpful too. There can be so much strain put on all family members when a major illness strikes. Each person may hide strong but similar feelings from one another. With effective help and willingness, relationships can grow stronger. Opening the channels for honest discussion and clarifying needs and feelings has united many families in the quest for healing. Facing feelings and problems courageously and honestly can be challenging. However, many families who have sought counseling report even more fulfilling lives than before they had to cope with cancer.

Fear of cancer recurrence is normal, but extreme and unrealistic fears may immobilize people. Asking the questions you need answered to ease your worry is warranted. There really are no stupid questions. It is best not to expend energy in worry that you could use more wisely in caring for yourself. Talking about your feelings with a family member or friend, your physician, or support group can help you deal with troubling concerns and emotions. Let others know you need help.

Nutrition and Diet

How we feel emotionally can certainly be influenced by how well we nourish our bodies physically. Balanced nutrition is important. When it comes to cancer, there are a number of important considerations and controversies regarding diet.

Most of the information on diet and cancer in mainstream medicine is limited to *preventing* cancer. Unfortunately, there is little in the way of mainstream medical advice regarding specific nutritional strategies for *treating* cancer. When a patient with cancer asks a physician about specific dietary recommendations, he/she will probably be told to "eat whatever you want as long as you keep your weight up." But there are other important considerations.

Doctors call fat, protein, and carbohydrates—the three main types of nutrients in food—*macronutrients.* Studies of the diets of diverse populations throughout the world suggest a correlation between the amount of fat in the diet and the incidence of cancer. Studies of specific populations in the United States, such as women with breast cancer, have yielded conflicting results regarding the role of dietary fat in cancer. Ongoing trials of low-fat dietary interventions should define the relation between fat intake and cancer risk. It is considered prudent to follow this dietary recommendation now, given the evidence that fat intake is related to heart disease as well as the possible link to cancer. This would seem to be a low-risk strategy for the patient with cancer, so long as normal weight is maintained.

> *Relaxation techniques and imagery has really helped me to manage my pain. I imagine myself lying on a beach and my pain washes away with the rhythm of the waves.*
>
> *Denise, 56*
> *Patient*

Micronutrients include vitamins and antioxidants. Available evidence suggests that some micronutrients are associated with a decreased risk of developing cancer while others are associated with an increased risk. Patients should be careful when taking these nutrients. Studies suggest that taking a multivitamin is important to provide a normal level of vitamins and minerals. Make sure that your multivitamin contains *selenium.* This micronutrient has antioxidant properties and may enhance the immune system. Previous trials in humans have raised the possibility that supplemental selenium is associated with a decreased occurrence of lung cancer. Additional trials hopefully will determine whether selenium reduces the incidence of new or second lung cancers in these patients.

There is strong evidence from a number of studies that eating fruits and vegetables lowers the risk of developing lung cancer. This observation and other data led to the theory that beta-carotene and/or vitamin A in these foods is the protective compound. However, neither supplemental beta-carotene nor vitamin A has been shown to lower the risk of developing lung cancer. In one large, well-done clinical trial, supplemental beta-carotene seemed to increase a smoker's risk of developing lung cancer. A recent analysis of this trial suggests that vitamin E (alpha-tocopherol) supplements might be beneficial in preventing lung cancer. Exercise caution when adding micronutrients to your diet. Although vitamins may help prevent certain cancers and are useful during recovery from cancer, experts warn against taking them during cancer treatments (chemotherapy or radiation). Many treatments work by depleting the tumor of nutrients it needs to grow.

Weight should be kept as close to normal as possible for both cancer prevention and treatment. The results of restrictive diets (calorie restriction or restriction of specific micronutrients) that claim to starve a tumor while supporting normal cells are unknown and not recommended. Alcohol should be consumed in moderation for cancer prevention.

I used art as a coping tool for myself, and then other people starting asking for it because it's motivational. We get so caught up with statistics, charts and graphs. Art is another way to send a message.

Sue, 42
Survivor

12

Complementary and Alternative Medicine

Some patients may wish to explore alternative therapies currently considered outside the mainstream of medical cancer treatment. Most cancer specialists accept that some of these therapies can improve the well-being and quality of life for someone with lung cancer, but evidence that these treatments can lengthen one's life is lacking. The most common alternative therapies are examined in this chapter.

The National Institutes of Health has adopted the term *complementary and alternative medicine* (CAM) for these treatments. However, a more descriptive term may be *integrative medicine*. Options reviewed here should be used in addition to but not as replacements for mainstream medical treatments. That is, they should be integrated into current cancer care. Clearly, patients should ask the same questions about these treatments that they would about mainstream treatments.

- How could the therapy help me? Could it be dangerous?

- Does the treatment operate according to known principles?
- Does any scientific literature support the use of the therapy?
- What is the practitioner's training? What are his/her claims regarding outcomes? Is the practitioner willing to make data available to open-minded investigators?
- What is the practitioner's reputation among peers?
- Does the practitioner encourage patients to reject conventional therapies that offer scientifically documented evidence of cure or significant improvement?

Note that scientific evidence of effectiveness may be lacking for certain treatments, such as energy work, healing touch, visualization, and prayer. However, it is difficult to imagine how any of these methods could harm someone. Today, many mainstream medical practitioners take their patients' interest in other therapies very seriously. Likewise, practitioners of the many alternative approaches have an obligation to work with those in mainstream medicine.

Psychological Approaches

Relaxation

For many, *progressive muscle relaxation* and biofeedback, a deep relaxation technique, are helpful. Progressive muscle relaxation involves moving your attention through all parts of your body with the instruction to let go of tension and tightness and relax more deeply. For some, these techniques can help decrease the nausea and vomiting related to chemotherapy, alleviate pain, and decrease the anxiety that often accompanies certain medical treatments. Music therapy can also be combined with progressive muscle relaxation to decrease anxiety and discomfort. Art therapy is a service that is more frequently being offered to patients. Painting, drawing, and creating are other ways of expressing feelings that can be very therapeutic. Ask your doctor if these services are available, or ask for a referral to a psychotherapist or a *psycho-oncologist*. Psycho-oncology is the study of psychological factors and their effects on cancer.

Hypnotherapy and Mental Imagery

My philosophy is that as long as patients feel like alternative therapies are helping, and the remedies are not hurting them, then it's a great complement to their therapy.
Scott, 49
Oncologist

Hypnotherapy focuses on identifying stressful situations in your life and desensitizing you to them. It may also teach better communication skills, expand effective coping skills, and foster relaxation. Look for a licensed or certified hypnotherapist with training in medical hypnotherapy.

Mental imagery plays a large part in these treatments. Some approaches help you envision the cancer cells being destroyed and the treatment being powerfully effective in helping your body repair itself. Other approaches help you connect with your own "wise self" or "inner voice" to visualize a desired outcome. Mental imagery can be a subtle but powerful technique.

Affirmations

Our beliefs influence how we view the world, relate to others, and behave generally. Affirmations are positive statements that when repeated can help change some of our conscious and unconscious programming. They are often used in other therapies but can be implemented alone. They are best stated with "I" in the present tense with an ideal feeling or outcome intended. You can begin with breathing. Breathe in life, love, joy, and peace. Exhale any tension or negativity. Then repeat one of the following affirmations that means the most to you, or use one of your own:

- I am at peace. I am worthwhile.
- I am vitally healthy.
- I deserve to be healed.
- I can be healed.
- I deeply love and accept myself as I am.
- I release all fears. I trust in the process of life.

Spiritual Approaches

A journey through illness often prompts deeper soul searching and spiritual exploration. Spiritual approaches to cancer include prayer, laying on of hands, and many forms of spiritual imagery or inner dialogue. Some define spirituality as having a deep relationship with the self. These approaches can definitely help you rediscover what is really valuable and meaningful. Recommit to making your dreams, joys, and passions come alive again. In so doing, you can move beyond feeling helpless to feeling empowered, helping both yourself and others along the way. Using our life experiences and wisdom to help others takes us beyond our personal concerns and reminds us that we have something of value to offer the world. Achieving deeper levels of self-awareness can decrease the stress of living with cancer. Cultivating inner peace, tranquility, and joy can bring balance, emotionally and physically. All of this can help in healing.

Spiritual approaches to cancer partially overlap religious approaches. One can be spiritual without being religious, and one can be religious without being spiritual. However, church affiliation has been shown to be instrumental in healthy outcomes. Ministers, rabbis, chaplains, and other spiritual advisors are often part of the hospital staff and can offer guidance.

Whatever will promote a renewed sense of enthusiasm in your life is vitally important now. Patients who face imminent death share poignant stories about the healing they received after being diagnosed with cancer. Healing, unlike curing of disease, may mean a transformation in how they live the rest of their lives. This can result in living with deeper meaning, allowing for the healing of old emotional wounds, repairing relationships, and feeling gratitude for all parts of life as one begins to understand the greater purpose of it all.

Keeping a Journal

Many people find that writing down their thoughts and experiences is very helpful. Keeping a journal is an excellent way to release emotional stress and develop a positive outlook. In a study of patients with asthma or rheumatoid arthritis, those who wrote on emotional topics experienced a reduction in symptoms, unlike those who did not keep a journal. Writing about your feelings about having lung cancer may help unlock further healing mechanisms for you. What would *you* write about? Often people have theories about why they got cancer. What is your theory? What are your unique gifts and talents? What do you think your contribution or purpose in life has been so far? How are you expressing the best of you?

Sometimes our losses and disappointments in life have not been fully grieved. Our hurts keep us closed and restricted. Give yourself permission to feel the sadness in order to let it go. Ask yourself what else do I need to let go of? What part of me needs attention? What do I really yearn for? What have I always wanted to do? What do I love and appreciate? How can I nurture myself more? Where do I need to be more gentle and patient with myself? What has stood in my way? What dreams do I wish to fulfill? What changes am I guided to make in my life by this illness?

Physical Approaches

Exercise

There are few if any studies of the effect of exercise on cancer patients. Most of the data are from preventive studies. Generally, these studies have shown that moderate exercise beginning later in life may decrease cancer risk. Some studies have failed to find this protective effect, however. Exercise has been shown to have a positive effect on depression, and this may benefit patients through one of the mind-body pathways. As noted earlier, a patient's performance status is related very closely to outcome. That is, patients in the best condition seem to do the best with treatment.

> *Exercise is a tremendous addition to people's lives. It helps patients to recover both physically and mentally.*
>
> *George, 41*
> *Physical Therapist*

Massage

Massage has a profoundly relaxing effect on people and is useful as a stress reliever. Areas of chronic pain can be relieved in many instances. One theoretical concern with cancer patients is that massage may stimulate lymphatic spread of certain cancers. Programs that use massage for people with cancer recommend that only gentle techniques be used in areas of known cancer activity. Massage therapists should avoid pressure in the areas of bone metastases. However, gentle back massages should not be a problem for most lung cancer patients. Still, patients should inform their massage therapists of any sensitive or painful areas, such as skin changes from radiation therapy.

Chiropractic Care

> *Just being there is the best thing that families and friends can do.*
>
> *Evelyn, 75*
> *Wife of Patient*

Chiropractors are usually aware that neck or spinal pain in a patient with lung cancer may be caused by spread of the cancer to the skeleton. Spinal manipulation in this setting could be dangerous. A patient with lung cancer should tell the chiropractors of the diagnosis before seeking treatment for neck or back pain. At the very least, chiropractic treatment should be coordinated with the patient's other cancer specialists, or perhaps avoided altogether.

Yoga

Yoga involves gentle stretching, breathing practices, and deep relaxation. On a physical level, yoga provides significant stress relief. However, practitioners of yoga also derive spiritual and psychological benefits from their practice. Yoga leads to a deep inner peace that serves to heal us at many levels. Yoga classes are offered in most cities and through universities and health clubs. Video tapes and books offer the beginner a way to start without access to a formal class. It is important never to strain or hold a position if it is uncomfortable. Therefore, it is especially important for patients with physical limitations to begin yoga with an experienced instructor who can demonstrate effective, alternative positions to the classically described ones.

Traditional Chinese Medicine

The World Health Organization (WHO) classifies the healing practices derived from ancient practices as *traditional medicine.* There are many forms of traditional medicine, but perhaps the one best known in the West is traditional Chinese medicine.

Traditional Chinese medicine includes acupuncture, Qi gong ("Qi" pronounced "Chee"), and herbal medicine. These methods manipulate the life force, or vital energy, which flows along body pathways called *meridians.* Each pathway is associated with a specific organ or body system. Practitioners consider disease to result from deficiency or imbalance of energy in the meridians and their associated physiological systems. Traditional Chinese medicine uses an intricate system of pulse and tongue diagnosis, palpation of points and meridians, medical history, and other signs and symptoms to diagnose a patient. A treatment plan is then formulated to restore the body to a balanced state of health. Most practitioners see their treatments as complementary to Western medicine, not replacements for it.

Sometimes I wonder if the people in lab jackets are just telling me things to make me feel more comfortable about a procedure. It's more believable to hear it from patients who have actually gone through it, but the health professionals are usually right.

Frank, 50
Patient

Acupuncture and Qi Gong

Acupuncture points are specific sites along the meridians. These points affect the flow of Qi. Practitioners can manipulate the flow of Qi with acupuncture needles or by exerting pressure on these points (*acupressure*). Patients have reported that acupuncture can relieve chemotherapy-related nausea and vomiting, chronic pain, even anxiety. Practitioners of Qi gong use movement and meditation to influence the flow of the vital energy. They claim to be able to feel the Qi (a sensation of warmth) and to be able to move it throughout the body. Millions of Chinese perform this "moving meditation" for one hour daily to promote health and peace of mind.

> *A lot of patients are interested in alternative therapies; however, we don't have strong scientific evidence to make recommendations. Use caution and inform your doctor about all medications, herbs and vitamins you are taking.*
> *Shelley, 37*
> *Nurse*

If you are interested in these therapies, find a practitioner who has been comprehensively trained in acupuncture and Oriental medicine. In the United States, over thirty states have established regulations or statutes for the practice of acupuncture. In these states, you should seek a licensed, registered or certified acupuncturist. Alternatively, you should find an individual in a nearby state who is licensed, or find a practitioner who is certified by the National Certification Commission for Acupuncture and Oriental Medicine (NCCAOM).

Herbals

Chinese herbal medicine is perhaps the main component of Oriental medicine. Published reports claim that it is effective in treating certain types of cancer. Judged by Western standards, however, these studies do not support the use of Chinese herbal medicine for cancer treatment. Patients should use herbal preparations and plant extracts with caution. There is a risk of harmful interactions with other medications. These preparations contain many potentially active ingredients, and the way they are made is often not standardized. Therefore, it is hard to know from one pill to the next just how much of the active ingredient is present. At a minimum, inform your mainstream medical doctor that you are taking herbal treatments. Check with a cancer specialist to make sure that there are no potentially harmful effects of combining herbal treatments with mainstream treatments. Medical doctors may not be aware of all of the ingredients in a specific preparation, but they should be willing to try to find out.

There are too many unconventional treatments to hope to review them all in this chapter. Those discussed here are the unconventional therapies that may be the most commonly considered ones.

13

Smoking: It's Never Too Late to Quit

Many people who develop lung cancer continue to smoke after diagnosis. Why quit now? Continuing to smoke increases the likelihood of developing complications from standard lung cancer treatments—surgery, chemotherapy and radiation therapy. Following surgery, smokers more often suffer lung problems such as pneumonia. They generally have more mucous to cough up afterwards and may have a more difficult time doing so. They may have to spend more time on a ventilator or in the hospital. Remember that survival after chemotherapy is closely related to one's performance status. Smoking may also worsen chemotherapy-related nausea and fatigue. It may decrease appetite and therefore impair nutrition. A similar logic applies to radiation therapy. Anything that a patient can do to improve his/her level of functioning helps. Anything that makes breathing harder—like smoking—doesn't help.

Preventing Other Diseases

Continuing to smoke increases the risk for other diseases. Smoking also causes heart disease, stroke and emphysema. With regard to heart disease, the good news is that the beneficial effects of quitting smoking are almost immediate. Tobacco smoke contains *carbon monoxide*, the same gas found in automobile exhaust, which binds to the body's red blood cells in place of oxygen. This deprives the heart and the rest of the body of oxygen at a time when it is most needed. Other compounds in tobacco smoke cause blood platelets to become stickier, increasing the likelihood of blood clots. If harmful clots form in the blood vessels that carry oxygen to the heart muscle, a heart attack may occur. If a clot forms in a blood vessel in the brain, a stroke may occur. Quitting smoking immediately lowers carbon monoxide levels in the blood, and the platelets begin to function more normally.

Smoking can cause emphysema, a progressive loss of functional lung tissue. Progressive emphysema leads to breathlessness and severe "loss of wind." Quitting smoking dramatically slows the further loss of lung function.

Cancer treatments that are designed to kill cancer cells inevitably damage some normal lung tissues and other tissues as well. This is often true of surgery when some surrounding lung tissue must be removed in order to extract all of the cancer. This is also true of radiation therapy. New treatment plans minimize the amount of normal lung treated by the radiation beam, but some normal lung tissue is still damaged. Therefore, it makes sense to quit smoking and conserve as much functioning lung as you can. View smoking cessation as part of your cancer treatment. It increases your chance of controlling or eliminating the cancer entirely.

Finally, another important reason to quit smoking is to avoid developing a second lung cancer in another part of your lung or in the other lung. The precancerous changes that eventually turned into a cancerous tumor in one area may also be present in other parts of your lungs. Continued exposure may produce another cancer. Clinical experience shows that a patient with a successfully treated early (stage I or II and some stage III) lung cancer has a 2-3 percent chance per year of developing another lung cancer. If the patient continues to smoke, the chance of developing a second lung cancer is even greater. Caring for your body isn't just limited to the period of time that you are receiving chemotherapy, radiation therapy, or surgery. It's a commitment to doing what is best for you for the rest of your life.

Choosing a Smoking Cessation Program

Millions of former smokers have successfully quit smoking by themselves. However, a patient with cancer has a lot to deal with already and may appreciate help from a smoking cessation program. The best results are generally obtained by participating in a comprehensive program, one that includes all the components currently recommended by the U.S. Agency for Health Care Policy and Research (AHCPR). Such a comprehensive program includes behavioral, addictive disorder, and relapse-prevention approaches. Smoking cessation specialists recognize that tobacco use is a complex behavior.

Choose a program that emphasizes how to change your behavior and consider seeing a counselor to support you. Ideally both individual counseling and support groups should be available. Drug therapy is an important component of a smoking cessation program. Although some forms of nicotine replacement therapy are available over the counter, specialists can prescribe certain forms and dosages not generally available to the public. Individualized doses of nicotine replacement drugs and combinations of drugs have proved effective in helping smokers quit but should only be used with medical supervision.

A Plan to Quit

Whether you participate in a comprehensive program or go it alone, quitting smoking is up to you. There is no "correct" way to quit smoking. Still, most people find it helps to do a little planning. Some people can simply make the decision to quit and never touch tobacco again. Smoking cessation experts do recommend picking a "quit date" at some point in the near future. Whether you decide to gradually smoke fewer cigarettes until that day and then quit or whether you smoke until that day and then go "cold turkey" is a matter of choice. Many smoking cessation clinics actually recommend the cold turkey approach.

> *I used medication to help me quit. It really took away the effects of withdrawal. I don't missing smoking at all!*
> *Jack, 45*
> *Former smoker*

Resisting the intense desire to smoke is difficult. Remember that this desire usually lasts only three to five minutes. Experts recommend coming up with a list of things to do other than smoking when your craving hits. Take a walk if you can, drink water, do some breathing exercises, or practice stress management. Suck on some hard candy, "puff" on a straw, keep your hands busy. Whatever works for you.

Don't be surprised if you crave cigarettes long after you quit smoking. Smoking is a complex behavior that involves more than simply the body "missing" nicotine. Most patients with lung cancer smoked for many years. It was probably an important part of your life, too. Spend a few minutes thinking about what you liked about smoking—it was great with that first cup of coffee, it was relaxing, or soothing, or it relieved boredom. Also list what you didn't like—coughing, expense, bad breath. Also think about when you smoked during a typical day. Try to identify what specific events made you crave a cigarette. Did you like to smoke while talking on the telephone, or after a meal, or after an argument with someone? Did a smoke break give you time to talk to friends at work? Once you have identified some of these smoking triggers, you can then think about how to respond when they come up in the course of daily life. Tell your friends that you are trying to quit, and that you'll visit with them later. You might try sipping bottled water while talking on the phone. These strategies can increase your chances of success.

If smoking is an underlying cause of lung cancer, why does the government continue to support its use? Smoking kills 400,000 people every year.
Betty, 50
Patient Advocate

Many smokers say they smoke to relieve stress. Others smoke to cope with underlying depression. Your doctor may be willing to prescribe medication to help with anxiety or depression. Few things in life are as stressful and emotionally difficult as a diagnosis of cancer. Participation in a support group or smoking cessation program can be of enormous benefit.

Once you have quit, reward yourself. Remaining a nonsmoker requires effort, sometimes for quite a while. It is different for every person. However, smoking cessation experts emphasize that most people make more than one serious attempt before actually quitting for good. It is important not to be discouraged by an occasional "slip" or even by smoking as before. Try to understand what caused you to want to smoke. See if you can handle that situation differently next time. Set another quit date and try again.

Many smokers first resolve to quit while they are in the hospital following surgery or for some other reason. It is an excellent time to quit. You are certainly in a supportive environment. The doctors and nursing staff are available to answer your questions and to monitor your use of nicotine patches or other prescriptions. It is still probably easier to not smoke while in the hospital than it will be at home. The hospital is a different environment without all the smoking triggers that you are accustomed to. Take some time while in the hospital to identify any smoking triggers that exist in your life. Decide how you will handle them effectively.

You never think it's going to happen to you, but when I was diagnosed with lung cancer, it was a real wake-up call. After smoking for 20 years, I quit cold turkey. I've been a nonsmoker for four years.

William, 41
Survivor

When You Decide to Quit

- Set a definite quit date.
- Dispose of all tobacco, lighters, ash trays.
- Let someone else know about your plan.
- Ask your doctor about medications that can help treat nicotine withdrawal. Learn how to use them.
- Be prepared to handle cravings and to feel discomfort for the first week or two.
- Expect to be less productive. Plan a lighter workload.
- Avoid situations that trigger smoking.

- Have low-calorie snacks available.
- Quit for one day at a time.
- Reward yourself for your success.
- If you slip, don't get discouraged.

Drug Therapy to Help Smokers Quit

Drug therapy plays an important role in a smoking cessation program. The two main classes of drugs are *nicotine replacement agents* and *bupropion,* also known as *Zyban.*

Nicotine has been identified as the addictive compound in tobacco smoke. Cigarettes, cigars, and chewing tobacco are basically nicotine delivery devices. The nicotine in tobacco is absorbed into the bloodstream and reaches the brain in literally seconds. There it stimulates the release of chemicals that in turn stimulate areas of the brain including the pleasure-related centers. Removing nicotine causes the various symptoms of withdrawal such as irritability, craving nicotine, and difficulty concentrating. Therefore, nicotine replacement therapy is designed to ease these symptoms and promote abstinence. Numerous studies have shown that those using nicotine replacement therapy have more success in kicking the habit.

Nicotine Gum

Nicotine replacement therapy comes in several forms. *Nicotine polacrilex,* better known as *nicotine gum,* was perhaps the first nicotine replacement therapy offered over the counter. It is used differently than regular gum. Patients should chew nicotine gum slowly until they feel a mild tingling, which is the nicotine being released. They should then "park" it between the cheek and gums for several minutes before chewing it again. This technique provides for gradual absorption and should continue for 30 minutes per piece of gum. Nicotine gum is available in 2-milligram and 4-milligram doses. Most patients find that 10 to 15 pieces per day are initially needed to successfully quit smoking.

Nicotine Patches

The *nicotine patches* are easier to use and deliver a continuous level of nicotine through the skin. The standard dose of 21 milligrams may not be enough for some heavy smokers. Patients should not exceed the recommended dose unless supervised by a physician. Side effects include mild skin irritation at the site of the patch. The directions recommend choosing a different, hairless site somewhere above the waist when placing a new patch.

Lung cancer has claimed the lives of four of my friends. They were all smokers. Quit smoking and encourage others to do the same. By advocating change, you can make a difference.
Robert, 55
Friend

Nicotine Nasal Spray

Like the gum, *nicotine nasal spray* must be used correctly for best results. The medication should be sprayed against the lower nasal lining where the nicotine is absorbed. It should not be sprayed or sniffed into the upper nasal passages. One spray into each nostril equals one dose (1 milligram). Patients should begin with 1 or 2 doses per hour, not to exceed 5 doses per hour. Most patients use about 15 doses per day. Gradually decrease the number of doses over time. Initially, most patients use 1 or 2 canisters per week. More than 2 canisters per week should not be used without medical supervision. Nasal irritation is a common initial side effect but diminishes with time. Most patients can use the spray successfully for up to 12 weeks.

Nicotine Inhaler

A *nicotine inhaler* has also proved effective in helping smokers quit. It may be the best choice for patients who need the ritual or "feel" of smoking that this device provides. Unlike a nicotine patch, which delivers a constant level of nicotine, an inhaler produces a more rapid increase and subsequent decrease in blood levels of nicotine, more like an actual cigarette. The device, although called an inhaler, is actually a "puffer." It resembles a cigarette holder and contains a small capsule filled with nicotine-treated cotton. Puffing on the device delivers vaporized nicotine to the lining of the mouth and upper throat, where it is absorbed. About 80 puffs over 20 minutes are required to obtain 2 milligrams of nicotine. The recommended daily dose is at least 6 capsules, up to 16 capsules.

> *Everyone has hurdles to jump in life. Lung cancer may be an obstacle, but I don't let it stand in the way of what is most important to me, my family.*
>
> Charles, 71
> Patient

Bupropion (Zyban)

Sustained-release bupropion, whose trade name is *Zyban*, is also an antidepressant. It is the first FDA-approved medication for smoking cessation that does not contain nicotine. It helps to stimulate the release of the same brain chemicals as nicotine, plus some others. These chemicals improve alertness, concentration, and memory. Bupropion also acts to prolong the effect of some of the brain chemicals that were previously stimulated by nicotine. In this sense, it can stimulate the pleasure centers and replace the effect of nicotine.

Bupropion is effective by itself for helping smokers quit. Therapy begins with 150 milligrams taken by mouth every morning for 3 or 4 days. If there are no intolerable side effects, a second 150 milligram dose per day is added. Doses should be taken at least 8 hours apart. Because one of the side effects of bupropion is insomnia, the second dose should be taken by late afternoon or early evening. Patients are usually instructed to continue smoking for the two weeks of therapy to allow a level of bupropion to build up before the planned quit date. Other possible side effects are a dry mouth and agitation. Seizures have been reported to occur in 1 out of every 1,000 patients. Therefore, patients with any of the following should not take bupropion:

- active seizures
- history of seizures
- previous head injury, stroke, brain surgery, or other injury that caused loss of consciousness
- use of drugs that lower the threshold for seizures (alcohol, neuroleptic agents)
- eating disorders (bulimia, anorexia nervosa)
- concurrent use of bupropion (in the form *Wellbutrin)* for depression
- use of monamine oxidase inhibitors, another class of antidepressants

Quitting smoking will significantly improve the quality of your life. Ask your doctor for help. Find out if there is a smoking cessation program in your hospital, cancer center, or community that you can join.

14

End-of-Life Care

E*nd-of-life care* is given to patients with advanced or terminal illnesses. Many of us will be involved in decisions about end-of-life care, either for ourselves or our loved ones. Complex decisions about life-sustaining treatments are difficult to make under any circumstances. Yet most people do not discuss these matters with their loved ones or with their doctors until they are seriously ill, often not even then.

If you've been diagnosed with an illness that could eventually take your life, take some time to consider issues that are important to you. For example, you may wish to consider the setting in which care will be delivered. There are also relevant legal and medical issues surrounding end-of-life care. Dealing with them now may make the process easier for both you and your loved ones.

Advance Directives

An *advance directive* is a written set of instructions in which you state your choices for future medical care. Living wills, health-care proxies, and durable power of attorney are all types of advance directives.

A *living will* provides instructions to your family, caregivers, and doctors about the types of medical care you wish to receive should you become incapacitated or unable to communicate your wishes. The living will removes the burden of making these decisions on your behalf from your family, friends, and physicians. Every patient has the right to accept or refuse specific medical treatments. Cancer Care, Inc., a nonprofit organization that provides information, assistance, and support for cancer patients, lists the following forms of life-sustaining therapy that you might want to consider when developing a living will:

- use of life-sustaining equipment (dialysis machines, respirators)
- "do not resuscitate" (DNR) orders, instructions not to use cardiopulmonary resuscitation
- CPR if breathing or heartbeat stops
- decision to provide or withhold fluids and nutrition provided by a tube or into a vein
- organ and tissue donations
- palliative (comfort) care

Communicate your wishes regarding end-of-life care to your family and doctors. Explaining your feelings and your values will protect you from having medical treatments imposed on you. Most states require that you have the document witnessed. Selecting comfort care over curative treatment means that you may still request antibiotics, pain medication, or other treatments. Your living will (or any advance directive) can be modified as your situation changes. You can change your mind at any time.

Check the specific guidelines in your state regarding a living will. You do not need a lawyer to draw one up. Forms can be obtained from hospitals, governmental offices on aging, legal offices, and organizations such as Choice in Dying (1-800-989-9455). Make copies of the living will and keep it in a safe place. Give additional copies to your doctor, hospital, and family.

A *health-care proxy* is a person whom you select to make medical decisions on your behalf if you cannot. Pick someone whose judgment you trust, and communicate to him/her your wishes for medical care beforehand. The *durable power of attorney* is the legal document that designates the person you choose. Have this document witnessed, notarized, and incorporated into your medical record.

We don't like to think about it, but people do die. That's why it's important to have affairs in order. Those who survive you need to know what to do. Spare everyone hassles and communicate with your family, regardless of your age.

Bridget, 48
Nurse

Settings for End-of-Life Care

Various settings are available for a patient's last months or days of life. The patient may live at home, in a nursing home or in a hospice setting. Whatever setting is chosen, the goal is the same: to keep the patient as comfortable as possible. Families facing end-of-life situations oftentimes use hospice services to assure the patient's comfort level.

Hospice Care

Hospice is a philosophy of care. The hospice treatment plan focuses on comfort control measures versus aggressive treatment for cure. Interdisciplinary team members develop treatment plans for each patient/family. Three types of support are provided:

Physical – with focus on pain and symptom control

Spiritual – to assist patient and family in prayer and coping with loss

Emotional – assessing coping strengths and possible need for additional support for patient and family

Hospice Team Members

- patient's family attending physician
- hospice medical director
- registered nurse (who advocates for symptom management)
- medical social worker (who provides community resource information and support)
- home health aide (who assists with hygiene)
- chaplain (for spiritual support and guidance)
- dietitian (who provides nutritional counseling)
- pharmacist (advocates for the patient regarding medications)
- volunteer coordinator (coordinates volunteer involvement on any level needed — respite, child care, transportation, meals)
- therapist (for physical, speech and occupational therapy as directed by the team)

- program coordinator (to oversee the team and assess progress of the hospice plans and goals)
- bereavement coordinator (who follows up with family after the patient is deceased)

Hospice care is "home centered" because the patient's family is the central part of the team. They provide most of the day-to-day care of the patient with the support of team members. In the United States, hospice services have traditionally been provided in the patient's home. However, there is a growing movement toward the development of "hospice houses" or "hospice floors" in nursing homes. They focus on providing a homelike environment.

Medicare pays for hospice services in the home. Medicare also pays for inpatient hospice care if the site is a Medicare-certified hospice facility. In these cases, Medicare pays for all services except the cost of room and board. More and more insurance companies are including hospice care in their coverage. Ask your insurance company about hospice coverage or ask your oncology social worker to investigate your insurance benefits on your behalf.

Appendix

Stage Grouping – TNM Designations for Non-Small Cell Lung Cancer

T = Tumor size   **N** = Lymph node involvement   **M** = Metastasis

Stage	TNM
0	Carcinoma in situ
IA	T1N0M0
IB	T2N0M0
IIA	T1N1M0
IIB	T2N1M0
	T3N0M0
IIIA	T3N1M0
	T1N2M0
	T2N2M0
	T3N2M0
IIIB	T4N0M0
	T4N1M0
	T4N2M0
	T1N3M0
	T2N3M0
	T3N3M0
	T4N3M0
IV	Any T Any N M1

TNM Descriptors

The following table provides a more thorough listing of TNM stages. The International Staging System for Lung Cancer describes the extent of spread of a malignant tumor according to the tumor-lymph node-metastasis (TNM) descriptions. The following is the most recently revised (1997) official version of the International Staging System for Lung Cancer.

Primary tumor (T)

TX   Primary tumor cannot be assessed, or tumor proven by the presence of malignant cells in sputum or bronchial washings but not visualized by imaging or bronchoscopy

T0   No evidence of primary tumor

Tis   Carcinoma in situ (malignant cells which have not deeply invaded tissue)

T1   Tumor greater than 3 cm in greatest dimension, surrounded by lung or visceral pleura, without bronchoscopic evidence of invasion more proximal than the lobar bronchus* (not in the main bronchus)

T2   Tumor with any of the following features of size or extent:
Greater than 3 cm in greatest dimension
Involves main bronchus, greater than 2 cm distal to the carina
Invades the visceral pleura
Associated with atelectasis or obstructive pneumonitis that extends to the hilar region but does not involve the entire lung

---

*   The uncommon superficial tumor of any size with its invasive component limited to the bronchial wall, which may extend proximal to the main bronchus, is also classified T1.

T3   Tumor of any size that directly invades any of the
following: chest wall (including superior sulcus tumors),
diaphragm, mediastinal pleura, parietal pericardium; or
tumor in the main bronchus less than 2 cm distal to the
carina, but without involvement of the carina; or associated
atelectasis or obstructive pneumonitis of the entire lung

T4   Tumor of any size that invades any of the following:
mediastinum, heart, great vessels, trachea, esophagus,
vertebral body, carina; or tumor with a malignant pleural or
pericardial effusion,** or with satellite tumor nodule(s)
within the ipsilateral primary tumor lobe of the lung

Regional lymph nodes (N)

NX   Regional lymph nodes cannot be assessed
N0   No regional lymph node metastases
N1   Metastasis to ipsilateral peribronchial and/or ipsilateral hilar
lymph nodes, and intrapulmonary nodes involved by direct
extension of the primary tumor
N2   Metastasis to ipsilateral mediastinal and/or subcarinal
lymph node(s)
N3   Metastasis to contralateral mediastinal, contralateral hilar,
ipsilateral or contralateral scalene, or supraclavicular lymph
node(s)

**   Most pleural effusions associated with lung cancer are due to tumor.
However, there are a few patients in whom multiple cytopathologic
examinations of pleural fluid show no tumor. In these cases, the fluid is
non-bloody and is not an exudate. When these elements and clinical
judgment dictate that the effusion is not related to the tumor, the effusion
should be excluded as a staging element and the patient's disease should be
staged T1, T2 or T3. Pericardial effusion is classified according to the same

Distant metastasis (M)

MX Presence of distant metastasis cannot be assessed
M0 No distant metastasis
M1 Distant metastasis present[***]

Stage grouping is the concept of combining subsets of patients classified according to TNM descriptors into categories called stages. These groupings are based on the fact that patients assigned to them have some common feature, such as a similar survival, or a similar response to current treatment. Representatives of the major international organizations of health professionals that treat patients with lung cancer meet periodically as necessary to revise the staging system to reflect new knowledge regarding the diagnosis, treatment, and outcome of patients with lung cancer.

[***] Separate metastatic tumor nodule(s) in the ipsilateral non-primary-tumor lobe(s) of the lung also are classified M1.

Resources

Cancer Care, Inc.
275 7th Ave.
New York, NY 10001
Phone: 212-302-2400 (1-800-813-HOPE)
www.cancercare.org
A nonprofit organization since 1944, Cancer Care offers
emotional support, information and practical help to people with
all types of cancer and their loved ones. All services are free.
Forty-five oncology social workers are available for phone
consultations in which they provide emotional counseling and
support; Cancer Care also offers education seminars,
teleconferences, and referrals to other services.

**Association for Lung Cancer Advocacy, Support, and Education
(ALCASE)**
1601 Lincoln Avenue
Vancouver, WA 98660
1-800-298-2436
www.alcase.org

This nonprofit organization is dedicated solely to helping those living with lung cancer improve the quality of their lives through advocacy, support, and education. The organization offers information on support groups as well as the "Phone Buddies" program, in which lung cancer patients are matched for a peer-to-peer support program.

American Cancer Society
599 Clifton Rd. NE
Atlanta, GA 30329-4251
Ph. 1-800-ACS-2345 (1-800-227-2345)
www.cancer.org
With more than two million volunteers and 3,400 local units, this organization works to eliminate cancer as a major health problem through prevention, saving lives and diminishing suffering through research, education, patient services, advocacy, and rehabilitation.

American Lung Association
1740 Broadway
NY, NY 10019
212-315-8700
Info@lungusa.org
http://www.lungusa.org
Founded in 1904 to fight tuberculosis, the organization today fights lung disease in all forms, with special emphasis on asthma, tobacco control, and environmental health.

University of Pennsylvania Cancer Center
http://www.oncolink.upenn.org
Well-respected site with useful links to other cancer-related sites.

Clinical Trials

Finding out if there is a clinical trial that you or a loved one might be eligible for can be a difficult task. Yet, it can be worth the effort. There are new trials and approaches devised all of the time, and it is difficult even for cancer specialists to keep up with all of them. One good place to start is by calling the toll-free Cancer Information Service of the National Cancer Institute 1-800-4-CANCER (1-800-422-6237); TTY at 1-800-332-8615. The Internet contains many listings of clinical trials at various sites. No specific site lists all of the available trials.

Cancer Care, Inc.
> http://www.cancercare.org
> This site also contains useful general information on clinical trials, including discussions of the pros and cons of participating, reimbursement issues, etc. It is written in an understandable format.

CenterWatch
> http://www.centerwatch.com
> A clinical trials listing service that provides information on private industry sponsored clinical trials as well as government-sponsored trials.

National Cancer Institute
> The Cancer Information Service provides information on clinical trials. Call 1-800-4-CANCER (1-800-422-6237); TTY at 1-800-332-8615. Visit CancerNet via the Internet. The URL is http://cancernet.nci.nih.gov. From there, one can access a database called PDQ, a computer system that provides updated information about cancer and cancer treatments. Cancer trials is a special section of the NCI website. The URL is http://cancertrials.nci.nih.gov

Internet Resources

Health information on the Internet, like most Internet content, is unregulated. That is, anyone is free to say or recommend whatever he/she wishes. The people behind medical web sites may have biases or may be advancing specific points of view. National medical organizations and some private groups have proposed guidelines and attempted to identify trustworthy sites. Adherence to these guidelines is voluntary, however. Therefore, it is up to users to be wary of medical claims and advice dispensed over the Internet. The best advice is to look first at information from government sites, educational sites, and non-profit organizations. These sites can be identified by the last part of their Internet addresses. Sites sponsored by the Federal government end in the suffix *.gov*. Those of university medical centers and other educational institutions end in *.edu*, and those of nonprofit organizations end in *.org*.

National Cancer Institute
> Bethesda, MD 20892
> Phone: (301) 496-4000
> Phone: 1-800-4-CANCER (1-800-422-6237)
> http://www.nci.nih.gov

National Heart, Lung & Blood Institute
> Bethesda, MA 20892
> http://www.nhlbi.nih.gov

National Center for Complementary and Alternative Medicine
> Bethesda, MD 20892
> http://www.nccam.nih.gov

U.S. Food and Drug Administration
FDA (HFE-88)
5600 Fishers Lane
Rockville, MD 20857
Phone: 1-888-INFO-FDA (1-888-463-6332)
http://www.fda/gov
Information about medications

Department of Health and Human Services
200 Independence Ave. S.W.
Washington, D.C. 20201
Phone: 1-877-696-6775 or (202) 619-0257
http://www.os.dhhs.gov

Healthfinder
http://www.healthfinder.gov
Consumer information from the U.S. Department of Health and
Human Services

Agency for Health Care Policy and Research (AHCPR)
2021 K St. NW
Washington, D.C. 20006
Phone: (202) 296-6922
Phone: 1-800-358-9295
http://www.ahcpr.gov

Centers for Disease Control and Prevention
1600 Clifton Rd.
Atlanta, GA 30333
Phone: (404) 639-3311
http://www.cdc.gov
The center provides statistics and other information about
diseases and conditions.

U.S. National Library of Medicine
8600 Rockville Pike
Bethesda, MD 20894
http://www.nlm.nih.gov

MEDLINE
>http://www.nih.gov/
>Produced by the National Library of Medicine, this site indexes articles from more than 3,500 medical journals. The service is aimed primarily at scientists and health professionals.

MEDLINEplus
>http://www.nlm.nih.gov/medlineplus
>Medline's site for the lay public.

Mayo Clinic Health Oasis
>http://www.mayohealth.org
>Mayo Clinic site includes disease and condition reports, health news and features, "Ask a Physician," library, and glossary.

InteliHealth
>http://www.intelihealth.com
>Johns Hopkins health information center features news and special reports, disease and condition guide, live chat, medical dictionary, physician locator, drug resource center and newsletter.

AMA Physician Select
>http://www.ama-assn.org
>From the American Medical Association, this site provides information on nearly every licensed physician in the United States.

HospitalSelect
>http://www.hospitalselect.com
>A hospital locator, providing information on virtually every hospital in the United States provided in cooperation with the American Medical Association.

Healthgrades
>http://www.healthgrades.com
>Profiles more than 500,000 hospitals and 600,000 physicians.

Resources

Medical Journals on Yahoo
http://dir.yahoo.com/Health/
Medicine/Journals links to numerous medical journals.

American Pain Society
http://www.ampainsoc.org
More than 3,200 doctors, nurses, scientists, psychologists, and pharmacologists who research and treat pain and act as advocates for patients in pain.

Mayday Pain Resource Center
http:mayday.coh.org
Pain resource center by City of Hope Medical Center, Duarte, CA.

HealthNewsDigest.com
News on health, science, technology and the environment.

WebMD
http://www.webMD.com
General health information. Features live chats with experts.

Drkoop.com
http://www.drkoop.com
Site affiliated with Dr. Everett Koop, former surgeon general. Features health news, resources, reports on health conditions and insurance information.

Mediconsult.com
http://www.Mediconsult.com
Comprehensive information on health conditions, live chat with experts, message boards.

DiscoveryHealth.com
http://discoveryhealth.com
Reports on health for men, women, seniors and children; health at work; nutrition; fitness; and weight control.

AccentHealth.com

http://www.accenthealth.com
Information on men's, women's and children's health; drugs;
nutrition. Features message boards, comprehensive list of
medical tests and procedures.

AllHealth.com

www.allHealth.com
Part of iVillage.network for women, this site offers reports on
health conditions, wellness and diet, news and special reports,
drug data base, chats with experts, message boards.

Hospice / End-of-Life Care

Choices in Dying

1035 30th Street, NW
Washington, DC 20007
Ph. (202) 338-9790
FAX: (202) 338-0242
www.choices.org
The inventor of living wills in 1967, this nonprofit organization is
dedicated to fostering communication about complex end-of-life
decisions. The organization provides advance directives,
counsels patients and families, trains professionals, advocates for
improved laws, and offers a range of publications and services.

National Hospice Organization (NHO)

1901 North Moore Street, Suite 901
Arlington VA 22209
(703) 243-5900
www.nch.org

Hospice Association of America

National Association of Home Care (NAHC)
228 Seventh Street, SE
Washington, DC 20003-4360
(202) 546-4759
www.hospice-america.org

Association of Oncology Social Workers
47000 Westlake Avenue
Glenview, IL 60025-1485
(847) 375-4721

American Academy of Hospice and Palliative Medicine
P.O. Box 14288
Gainesville, FL 32604-2288
(352) 377-8900
www.aahpm.org

Hospice Nurses Association
Medical Center East, Suite 375
211 North Whitfield Street
Pittsburgh, PA 15206-3031
(412) 361-2470
www.hpna.org

Smoking Cessation

Inquire about smoking cessation programs at your doctor's office, local hospital, or with local smoking cessation groups. Other ways to find programs close to home include contacting your state health department or your local branch of the American Cancer Society or American Lung Association.

American Lung Association offers a booklet, "Quit Smoking Action Plan." It offers specific recommendations for selecting a personalized plan to help you quit smoking. Write to them or visit the quit smoking action plan web site directly: www.lungusa.org/partner/quit/index.html. The American Lung Association's "7 Steps to a Smoke-Free Life" also offers sound advice on smoking cessation methods.

Glossary

A

Acupuncture: Traditional Chinese medical treatment that seeks to correct the flow of life force, or Qi, using thin needles placed at specific points on the body.

Adenocarcinoma: One type of non-small cell lung cancer that arises from mucous glands lining the air passages.

Adjuvant therapy: Therapy given after another, initial therapy.

Adrenal glands: Located on top of each kidney, these glands are one of the sites that lung cancer more commonly spreads to.

Advance directive: Legal document addressing the use of life support measures if required.

Affirmation: Positive statement that one says to oneself.

Alopecia: Hair loss.

Alternative medicine: Healing practices other than those of mainstream medicine.

Alveolus: Microscopic air sac in the lung where oxygen enters and waste gas exits the blood.

Analgesic: A substance that relieves pain.

Anemia: Low blood count.

Anesthesiologist: A physician who specializes in the administration of anesthesia.

Anhidrosis: An abnormal absence of sweat production on a certain area of the skin.

Anorexia: Loss of appetite for food.

Antiemetics: Drugs that are used to decrease the sensation of nausea.

Arterial blood gas: A blood test that provides information about lung function.

Asbestos: A mineral fiber formerly used in insulation that when inhaled increases the risk that a smoker can develop lung cancer.

B

Best supportive care: Treatment for advanced lung cancer aimed at decreasing symptoms caused by the cancer rather than destroying the cancer.

Biofeedback: Technique that provides a person with information about his/her physiologic state (level of relaxation, for example) with the goal of eventually learning to control that state.

Biopsy: Surgical removal of a portion or all of a mass or organ.

Bladder: Organ that collects urine from the kidneys.

Blood count: A test that counts the number of different cells that are contained in the blood.

Bone marrow: Tissue contained within the center of bones that makes the blood cells.

Bone scan: A test that can identify if cancer has spread to bone.

Brachytherapy: Radiation treatment that uses radioactive pellets inserted into a flexible tube placed inside the breathing passage to directly treat a lung cancer.

Brain: Contained in the skull and responsible for thought, the brain is also a site that lung cancer can spread to.

Breastbone: Flat bone on the front of the chest that the ribs connect to.

Bronchial basal epithelial cells: Cells that line the breathing passages, common site where lung cancers develop.

Bronchial tree: The multiple airways and their branches contained within the lungs.

Bronchoalveolar carcinoma: One specific type of non-small cell lung cancer that can be diffuse, multicentric or localized. If localized, surgical removal may be associated with a high cure rate.

Bronchoscope: Long, thin flexible or rigid tube used to look into the breathing passages of the lung.

Bronchus: The main or large breathing passage in each lung.

C

CPR: Cardiopulmonary resuscitation, a technique to revive a person after the heart has stopped.

Cancer: Tissue made up of cells that grow uncontrollably, invade other tissues and spread to other parts of the body.

Carbon dioxide: A by-product of normal body function, this waste gas is exhaled from the lungs.

Carcinogen: Any cancer-producing substance.

Carcinoma in situ: Cancer that is still confined to the area where it first developed.

CAT scan: Computerized axial tomography, or CT scan, an x-ray test that produces cross-sectional images of the body that are more detailed than standard x-rays.

Cell: The fundamental structural and functional unit of living organisms.

Cervical mediastinoscopy: A procedure during which a thin tube is inserted through an incision above the breastbone in order to examine tissue in the area between the lungs.

Chemotherapy: The treatment of a disease, such as cancer, with chemical agents.

Chest tube: A flexible tube inserted between the ribs and into the space surrounding the lungs in order to drain air or fluid.

Chest x-ray: A picture of the chest taken with x-rays.

Chiropractic: A field of healing based on spinal manipulation and alignment.

Chronic obstructive pulmonary disease: A name for a number of long-term breathing problems with various causes such as aging and smoking.

Clavicle: The collarbone.

Community Clinical Oncology Program (CCOP): A program funded by the National Cancer Institute designed to make clinical trials available to patients in community hospitals.

Complementary medicine: Healing practices other than those of mainstream medicine.

Complication: An undesired additional problem related to a disease process or to a treatment for a disease.

Computerized tomography: See CAT scan.

Counseling: Discussions with a health professional regarding assistance with life situations, behavior, relationships, and feelings.

Curative treatment: A treatment intended to eradicate disease.

D

Diagnose: To determine the cause of an illness or medical condition.

Diagnostic radiologist: A medical specialist trained to read x-rays.

Diaphragm: A muscle located between the chest and the abdomen that helps with breathing.

Diarrhea: Liquid or watery stool.

Diffusion capacity: A test that helps to determine the amount of functioning lung tissue.

Do not resuscitate orders (DNR): An order given that prevents medical personnel from reviving a person who stops breathing or whose heart stops beating.

Durable power of attorney: A legal document that gives a person or persons the authority to make decisions for another person.

Dysphagia: Difficulty swallowing either solids or liquids.

Dysplasia: An increase in both the number of cells in a tissue and in the size of those cells, a precancerous change.

Dyspnea: Shortness of breath.

E

Emphysema: A condition affecting the lungs characterized by loss of functioning lung tissue and progressive shortness of breath.

End-of-life care: Palliative and supportive care given to persons with a terminal illness.

Endorphins: Compounds made by the body that affect the perception of pain.

Esophagus: The muscular swallowing tube that connects the mouth and the stomach.

Excisional biopsy: Surgical removal of an entire mass in order to determine what it is.

Exercise treadmill test: A test that measures the heart and lung function of a person while they are walking on a treadmill.

Exploratory thoracotomy: Chest surgery that is performed when no clear preoperative diagnosis was possible.

Extensive disease: A term used to describe small cell lung cancer when it has spread beyond the chest.

External beam radiation therapy: Radiation therapy that is given by directing a beam of radiation at the cancer from a source located outside of the body.

F

Fatigue: A feeling of tiredness and lack of energy, related to cancer or cancer treatment or both.

Femur: The thigh bone.

Five-year survival: In the setting of lung cancer, this term is often synonymous with cure.

Food and Drug Administration (FDA): The federal government agency that is responsible for approving new medical treatments.

G

General anesthetic: A state of unconsciousness produced by anesthetic agents.

Glucose: A sugar that is the chief source of energy for living organisms.

Granulocyte colony stimulating factor (G-SF): A drug that stimulates the production of infection-fighting white blood cells.

H

Headache: Pain in the head, in certain settings could be sign of a brain metastasis.

Health-care proxies: A legal document that authorizes someone other than the patient to make decisions for the patient about health issues when necessary.

Hemoptysis: Coughing up any amount of blood.

Hemorrhoids: Veins near the anus that can become swollen and painful and sometimes bleed.

Hoarseness: Raspy voice.

Horner's syndrome: Symptoms (a small pupil, a droopy eyelid, and absence of sweating all on one side of the face) signifying dysfunction of the sympathetic nerve on that side of the body.

Hospice: A facility that provides supportive care to terminally ill patients and their families.

Hyperplasia: An abnormal increase in the number of cells in an otherwise normal tissue.

Hypnotherapy: The use of hypnosis in the treatment of disease.

I

Imagery: A technique that uses visualization for the purposes of healing.

Immunosuppressant: An agent that diminishes or prevents the immune response.

Incision: A wound made by cutting with a sharp instrument for the purpose of performing an operation.

Infection: Inflammation in body tissue caused by microorganisms.

Inflammation: A localized response to tissue injury characterized by swelling, redness, heat, tenderness, and loss of function.

Infusion: The therapeutic introduction of fluid or medicine into a vein.

Institutional review board: A group authorized to insure that research that involves humans is conducted according to ethical standards.

Integrative medicine: A term for the combined use of mainstream medical techniques with alternative medicine.

Interventional radiologist: A specialist trained to perform procedures, such as biopsies, using imaging equipment such as x-rays.

Intravenous: Administration of medication or fluid to a patient by introducing it through a vein.

J

K

L

Large cell carcinoma: A specific type of non-small cell lung cancer which may grow and spread more aggressively.

Laryngeal nerves: Nerves that activate the vocal cords.

Larynx: The voice box in the neck.

Lid lag: A droopy eyelid, one that moves more slowly when blinking.

Limited disease: A term that describes small cell lung cancer when it has not spread beyond the chest.

Liver: An organ located in the right upper part of the abdomen that has a number of important bodily functions. One of the organs that lung cancer can spread to.

Living will: A document indicating the treatments a person will accept or not accept for use in the event that they are unable to communicate those wishes.

Lobectomy: The surgical removal of one of the lobes of a lung.

Lobes: One of the main divisions of a lung.

Local anesthetic: A drug used to block sensation in a specific area of the body.

Low-dose spiral CT scan: A CT scan that uses fewer x-rays used for early lung cancer detection.

Lungs: The organs that supply the blood with oxygen and rid the body of carbon dioxide.

Lymph nodes: Collections of lymph tissue located throughout the body, they are a source of lymphocytes that fight infection and cancer.

M

Magnetic resonance imaging (MRI): A machine that produces images of the body using magnetic fields.

Malignant tumor: A tumor that can invade tissue, grow uncontrollably and spread to other tissues, a cancer.

Massage: A relaxation technique.

Mediastinal lymph nodes: Lymph nodes located in the chest between the lungs, common site of lung cancer spread.

Mediastinoscope: Thin tube inserted into the mediastinum that doctors look through in order to view this area, biopsy lymph nodes, etc.

Mediastinum: That area between the lungs that contains the heart, the windpipe, the esophagus, lymph nodes, nerves, and blood vessels.

Medical oncologist: A specialist trained to use medicine to treat cancers.

Metastasis: An area of cancer that has spread from another part of the body.

Microscope: An instrument that provides magnified images of very tiny objects.

Minimally invasive surgery: Surgery through small incisions, sometimes using television cameras to provide adequate vision for the surgeons.

Miosis: A smaller than normal (constricted) pupil.

Multimodality therapy: A treatment program that combines at least two of the three main methods for treating cancer surgery, radiation therapy or chemotherapy.

Mutation: A change in genetic material.

N

National Cancer Institute: U.S. government agency charged with promoting research and new treatment of cancer.

Nausea: A sensation of needing to vomit.

Needle biopsy: A procedure in which a needle is advanced through the chest into a tumor mass within or near the lung in order to obtain a small piece of the tumor.

Neoadjuvant therapy: Refers to treatments such as chemotherapy or combined chemotherapy and radiation therapy when they are given before surgical treatment.

Nerves: A fiber containing nerve cells that conveys impulses from the central nervous system to other parts of the body.

Neurologic: Referring to the nervous system.

Nicotine replacement therapy (NRT): Any of several methods of administering nicotine in order to minimize symptoms of withdrawal arising from smoking cessation.

Non-small cell lung cancer: The most common type of lung cancer, it accounts for 75-80% of all lung cancers.

O

Oncologist: A physician who specializes in the treatment of cancer patients.

Operation: A procedure performed by a surgeon to remove or repair part of the body.

P

PET: Positron emission tomography.

Palliative treatment: Treatment administered with the goal of making the patient feel better or to improve function as opposed to destroying a cancer.

Pancoast syndrome: A collection of symptoms including pain in the arm and in the armpit, wasting of the arm muscles, and Horner's syndrome caused by a lung cancer growing at the top of the lung.

Parietal pleura: The layer of tissue that lines the inside of the chest cavity.

Pathologist: A medical specialist trained to detect the structural changes in tissues and cells caused by disease.

Patient-controlled analgesia (PCA): A device that allows the patient to self-administer safe amounts of pain medication.

Performance status: A way of describing the overall function of a person, a key indicator of response to chemotherapy.

Perfusion scan: A test that estimates the blood flow to each lung.

Pericardium: The sac that surrounds the heart.

Peripheral neuropathy: Functional disturbances of the peripheral nerves sometimes caused by chemotherapy, accounting for symptoms such as numbness and tingling sensations in the hands and toes.

Peripheral vascular disease: Hardening of the arteries occurring in blood vessels other than the heart.

Phrenic nerve: The nerve responsible for moving the diaphragm muscle during breathing, there is one nerve on each side of the chest.

Platelets: Cells in the blood that are important for blood clotting.

Pleura: The layer of cells covering the lungs and the inside of the chest cavity, the pleura surrounds the pleural space.

Pleural effusion: Fluid that has accumulated in the pleural space surrounding the lungs.

Pleuritic chest pain: Sharp, stabbing chest pain that occurs with breathing.

Pneumonectomy: The surgical removal of an entire lung.

Pneumonia: An infection within the lung.

Pneumothorax: Air that has accumulated in the pleural space.

Port: A device usually implanted under the skin that is used for the infusion of drugs or fluid into the blood stream or for drawing blood for blood tests.

Positron emission tomography: A test that produces an image based on the uptake of glucose by a cancer, used to determine if a tumor is a cancer and if a cancer has spread.

Prognosis: The likely outcome of a disease, often given in terms of the expected chance of surviving for a certain number of years.

Progressive muscle relaxation: A relaxation technique.

Prophylactic cranial irradiation: Radiation therapy given to the brain in patients with small cell lung cancer to prevent brain metastases from developing.

Psycho-oncologist: A specialist in the psychological aspects of cancer.

Psychotherapist: A specialist who treats behavioral and mental disorders using a variety of methods other than the use of drugs.

Pulmonary artery: The blood vessel that brings blood that is depleted of oxygen to the lungs.

Pulmonary function tests: A general term for a number of breathing tests and blood tests that together measure lung function.

Pulmonary medicine specialist: A medical doctor trained in the diagnosis and treatment (with medicines) of lung and breathing disorders.

Pulmonary vein: The blood vessel that brings oxygenated blood from the lungs to the heart so that it can be pumped to the rest of the body.

Q

Qi: (pronounced "Chee") The Chinese word for "life force."

Qi gong: A Chinese martial art involving manipulation of Qi through movement and breathing.

Quit date: The date chosen to stop smoking entirely.

R

Radiation oncologist: A medical doctor specializing in the treatment of cancer with radiation.

Radiation recall: The reoccurrence of a side effect of radiation treatments (such as skin irritation) long after the radiation therapy has been completed.

Radiation therapist: A specially trained technician who administers radiation treatments.

Radiation pneumonitis: Inflammation in the lung that sometimes results from the radiation therapy beam.

Radioactive seeds: Small pellets of radioactive material that can be placed down a catheter positioned in the breathing passage during brachytherapy.

Radon: A naturally occurring gas originating from the ground that when inhaled is associated with increased rates of lung cancer development.

Red blood cells: The cells in the blood that carry oxygen.

Resectable: The finding that a cancer does not grow into any vital structure and can therefore be removed by a surgical procedure.

Respiratory therapists: Specially trained technicians who monitor and maintain the respiratory status of patients.

Rib: The bones of the chest wall that make the chest rigid, making breathing possible.

S

Screening: The detection of a disease process before it causes any symptoms.

Sedation: Medication given to reduce awareness.

Segments: Subdivisions of a lobe.

Segmentectomy: The smallest anatomically complete resection of the lung that can be performed.

Seizures: Convulsions or muscle spasms sometimes caused by spread of cancer to the brain.

Shortness of breath: The sensation of not being able to catch one's breath.

Side effects: A consequence of a treatment other than the one for which it was used.

Sign: Observable evidence of disease.

Small cell lung cancer: One of the two main types of lung cancer, often widespread by the time it is diagnosed.

Sputum: Material brought up from the breathing passages.

Sputum cytology: Analysis of cells present in sputum to determine if there are signs of cancer.

Squamous cell carcinoma: One of the specific types of non-small cell lung cancer.

Stage: The anatomic extent of a cancer, how far it has spread.

Staging: The methods and procedures in determining the stage of a cancer.

State-of-the-art: The most advanced and latest methods.

Stroke: Sudden loss of brain function from bleeding, blood clot, or other injury.

Subclavian vein: Large vein behind the clavicle, sometimes used for infusion of fluid or medicine.

Submucosal gland cells: Cells that line the breathing passages where adenocarcinoma arises.

Superior vena cava: The large vein that drains blood from the head, neck and arms back to the heart, may be blocked by a lung cancer in the upper right lung.

Superior vena cava syndrome: Swelling in the head, neck and arms caused by obstruction of the superior vena cava by a lung cancer.

Surgeon: A medical doctor trained to perform operations.

Survival: The act of continuing to live after a certain event, such as a diagnosis of lung cancer.

Symptom: A change in condition as perceived by a patient, subjective evidence of disease.

T

TNM: An abbreviation for tumor, lymph nodes, and metastases, a method of describing important features about a cancer.

Thoracic surgeon: A surgeon who has undergone at least two additional years of training in order to specialize in heart and lung surgery.

Thoracotomy: General term for an operation on the chest using an incision made between the ribs.

Three-dimensional conformal radiation therapy: A special method of treating someone with external beam radiation therapy that minimizes exposure of normal tissue to radiation.

Tissue: Body components made up of living cells.

Trachea: The windpipe.

Traditional chinese medicine: A system of healing based on concepts of vital energy and natural forces, the therapies consist of herbal remedies and methods of manipulating the vital force, Qi.

Transfusion: The procedure of giving blood or blood products to a person.

Transthoracic needle aspiration biopsy: The technique of sticking a needle through the chest and into the lung or mediastinum for the purpose of taking a biopsy of a tumor or other mass.

Tumor: Any mass or growth.

U

V

Very early stage disease: Description of small cell lung cancer identified as a localized, potentially resectable tumor.

Video-assisted thoracoscopy (VATS): Minimally invasive surgery on the chest using a special television camera and special instruments.

Visceral pleura: The lining on the surface of the lung.

W

Wedge resection: Removing a small piece of the lung, usually with a surgical stapler.

Wheezing: Noisy breathing as a result of a partially obstructed breathing passage.

White blood cells: Cells in the blood that fight infection.

Wound infection: Infection of a surgical incision.

X

Y

Yoga: Breathing and stretching discipline.

Z

Zubrod scale: Rating system describing the functional status of a person.

Index

About the Author

Walter Scott, M.D. is a board-certified cardio-thoracic surgeon and Associate Professor of Surgery and of Preventive Medicine and Public Health at Creighton University School of Medicine in Omaha, Nebraska. He specializes in the surgical treatment of lung cancer.

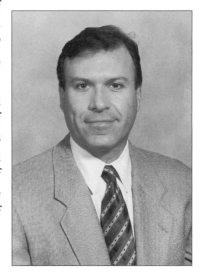

Dr. Scott's research interests include the use of positron-emission tomography (PET) to diagnose and stage lung cancer, the use of spiral CT screening to detect early lung cancer, and the use of minimally invasive surgical techniques.

Dr. Scott received his medical degree from the University of Chicago Pritzker School of Medicine in Chicago, Illinois. He completed his general surgical residency and fellowship in cardiothoracic surgery at the University of Chicago Hospitals. In 1992, Dr. Scott joined the faculty of the Creighton University School of Medicine.

Dr. Scott is a Fellow of the American College of Chest Physicians and co-chair of the Section on Lung Cancer. He is also a member of the Society of Thoracic Surgeons. Dr. Scott is a member of the Missouri Valley Community Clinical Oncology Program, the North Central Cancer Treatment Group, and the Thoracic Organ Committee of the American College of Surgeons Oncology Group. He serves as co-director of the Creighton Multidisciplinary Chest Tumor Clinic. Dr. Scott maintains a web site about lung cancer for physicians and the public at: www.lungcancer.creighton.edu.

Addicus Books Consumer Health Titles

Cancers of the Mouth and Throat—A Patient's Guide to Treatment   *$14.95*
William Lydiatt, MD and Perry Johnson, MD /
1-886039-44-5 (Fall 2000)

Coping with Psoriasis—A Patient's Guide to Treatment   *$14.95*
David L. Cram, MD / 1-886039-47-X (July 2000)

The Healing Touch—Keeping the Doctor/Patient   *$9.95*
Relationship Alive Under Managed Care
David L. Cram, MD / 1-886039-31-3

Hello, Methuselah! Living to 100 and Beyond   *$14.95*
George Webster, PhD / 1-886039-25-9

Living with P.C.O.S.—Polycystic Ovarian Syndrome   *$14.95*
A. Boss and E. Sterling / 1-886039-49-6

Lung Cancer—A Guide to Treatment & Diagnosis   *$14.95*
Walter J. Scott, MD / 1-886039-43-7 (April 2000)

Overcoming Postpartum Depression and Anxiety   *$12.95*
Linda Sebastian, RN / 1-886930-34-8

Prescription Drug Abuse—The Hidden Epidemic   *$14.95*
Rod Colvin / 1-886039-22-4

Simple Changes: The Boomer's Guide to a Healthier, Happier Life   *$9.95*
L. Joe Porter, MD / 1-886039-35-6

Straight Talk About Breast Cancer   *$12.95*
Suzanne Braddock, MD / 1-886039-21-6

The Stroke Recovery Book   *$14.95*
Kip Burkman, MD / 1-886039-30-5

The Surgery Handbook—A Guide to Understanding Your Operation   *$14.95*
Paul Ruggieri, MD / 1-886039-38-0

Understanding Parkinson's Disease: A Self-Help Guide   *$14.95*
David Cram, MD / 1-886039-40-2

Please send:

_____ copies of _____
(*Title of book*)

at $ _____each   TOTAL: _____

Nebr. residents add 5% sales tax   _____

Shipping/Handling
  $3.20 for first book.
  $1.10 for each additional book   _____

            TOTAL ENCLOSED: _____

Name_____

Address_____

City _____State _____Zip_____

       Visa   Master Card   Am. Express

Credit card number_____Expiration date _____

Order by credit card, personal check or money order. Send to:
Addicus Books
Mail Order Dept.
P.O. Box 45327
Omaha, NE 68145
Or
online at **www.AddicusBooks.com**